An Introduction to Cancer Care

An Introduction to Cancer Care

Tracey McCready BSc, RGN, HETC, ILTM
Lecturer, Public Health and Cancer Care Team, Faculty of Health and Social Care, University of Hull

Julie M MacDonald MSc, BSc, RGN, RM CertEd, ILTM
Lecturer, Care of the Older Person Team, Faculty of Health and Social Care, University of Hull

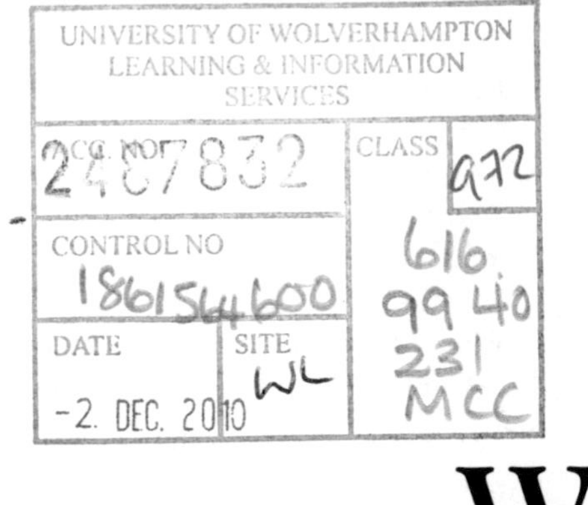

W
WHURR PUBLISHERS

The Atrium, Southern Gate, Chichester,
West Sussex PO19 8SQ, England
Telephone (+44) 1243 779777

Email (for orders and customer service enquiries): cs-books@wiley.co.uk
Visit our Home Page on www.wiley.com

Reprinted 2006

Other Wiley Editorial Offices

John Wiley & Sons Inc., 111 River Street, Hoboken, NJ 07030, USA

Jossey-Bass, 989 Market Street, San Francisco, CA 94103-1741, USA

Wiley-VCH Verlag GmbH, Boschstr. 12, D-69469 Weinheim, Germany

John Wiley & Sons Australia Ltd, 42 McDougall Street, Milton, Queensland 4064, Australia

John Wiley & Sons (Asia) Pte Ltd, 2 Clementi Loop #02-01, Jin Xing Distripark, Singapore 129809

John Wiley & Sons Canada Ltd, 22 Worcester Road, Etobicoke, Ontario, Canada M9W 1L1

Wiley also publishes its books in a variety of electronic formats. Some content that appears in print may not be available in electronic books.

A catalogue record for this book is available from the British Library

ISBN -13 978-1-86156-460-3 (PB)
ISBN -10 1-86156-460-0 (PB)

Printed and bound in Great Britain by TJ International Ltd, Padstow, Cornwall

This book is printed on acid-free paper responsibly manufactured from sustainable forestry in which at least two trees are planted for each one used for paper production.

Contents

Preface

> I need to know that you know that within my body there is me.
>
> Petrone (1999, p. 1)

The diagnosis and treatment of cancer can have a devastating impact on the lives of patients, their families and carers, bringing uncertainty and sometimes debilitating consequences of treatment. Support is needed for preventive strategies, diagnosis and treatment, and sometimes for palliative care (Department of Health or DoH 2000, National Institute for Clinical Effectiveness or NICE 2004).

A patient survey produced before publication of The NHS Cancer Plan (DoH 2000) highlighted the priorities of cancer patients: to be treated with humanity, dignity and respect; to enjoy good communication with health-care professionals; to have clear information about their condition and the different treatment options available; to receive the best possible symptom control; and to receive appropriate psychological support when necessary.

This book is written as an introductory text for those health-care professionals who wish to gain knowledge that will enable them to provide holistic care for patients and their families with cancer. Although not exhaustive, the text should be used as a guide.

A cancer diagnosis has a great impact both physically and psychologically not only on the patient but also on their families and carers. Care needs to be holistic and evidence based so that the patient can experience the best possible quality of life throughout the cancer journey. The structure of this book relates closely to this journey and also to national guidelines for excellence in cancer care.

The aim of the book is to take the reader on the cancer journey, starting with understanding of the nature of cancer, health promotion and screening and then moving on to explore the common cancers and treatments. Other topics covered include body image and sexuality, pain and symptom management, and ethical and legal issues. The final chapter explores aspects of surviving cancer. Research, communication skills and psychosocial care are themes that run throughout the book, together with multiprofessional working.

Although the book is designed to be read as a whole, each chapter can also stand alone, so the chapters can be read in any order. We believe that good communication skills, a good knowledge base and empathy are essential for the delivery of good quality cancer care.

Even when no treatment is available and a cure is not possible, understanding the meaning of the illness for the person and that person's life is, in itself, a form of healing, in that such understanding can overcome the sense of alienation and loss of self-understanding and social integration that accompany illness (Benner and Wrubel 1989).

Tracey McCready
Julie MacDonald
March 2005

References

Benner P, Wrubel J (1989) The Primacy of Caring: Stress and coping in health and illness. Los Angeles, CA: Addison-Wesley.

Department of Health (2000) The NHS Cancer Plan: A plan for investment, a plan for reform. London: HMSO.

National Institute for Clinical Effectiveness (2004) Improving Supportive and Palliative Care for Adults with Cancer: The manual. London: NICE.

Petrone MA (1999) Touching the Rainbow: Pictures and words by people affected by cancer. Brighton: East Sussex Health Authority.

Chapter 1

Understanding cancer

There are over 200 different types of cancer that can occur anywhere in the body, all having different causes and symptoms and all requiring different treatments (Cancer Research UK 2004). In the UK, the lifetime risk of developing cancer is one in three. Cancers affect people at different ages, with the risk rising significantly with age; 65% of cancers occur in people aged over 65 (Cancer Research UK 2004).

A cancer develops when a cell experiences a mutation that makes the cell divide more rapidly than usual, leading to an overgrowth of tissue (National Institutes of Health or NIH 2004). This overgrowth is often referred to as a tumour. Some tumours are not cancerous and are termed 'benign'; those tumours that are cancerous are termed 'malignant'. Uncontrolled growth of cells causes the tissue to look abnormal. If malignant cells are contained within the original tissue the cancer is called *in situ*, whereas if they invade neighbouring tissue the cancer is said to be invasive. One property of most malignant tumours is their ability to undergo metastasis – the spread of cancerous cells to other parts of the body (Tortora and Grabowski 2004).

Several factors may cause a cell to become cancerous, e.g. environmental agents in the food we eat, chemical agents, radiation and viruses. These agents are called carcinogens and cause mutations in the genetic make-up of the cell (Tortora and Grabowski 2004).

History of cancer and its treatment

The earliest description of cancer is from Egypt in the seventeenth century BC, when a physician wrote about a patient with cancer suggesting that there is no treatment. The *Edwin Smith Papyrus* describes tumours of the breast (American Cancer Society 2004).

In the fifth century BC, Hippocrates, the 'father of medicine', suggested in his writings that it is better not to apply any treatment in cases of occult (hidden) cancer because, if treated, the patients die quickly whereas if not treated the patient holds out for longer (Yarbro et al. 2000). It is a widely held belief that the word *karkinos*, Latin for crab, was first applied to cancer by Hippocrates. *Karkinos* aptly describes the appearance of a malignant tumour, which is irregular in outline and uncontained, because crabs move in an erratic manner, sideways, often with sudden bursts of movement (Morgan 2001).

The Egyptians blamed cancer on various gods. Hippocrates explained all diseases as resulting from an imbalance of the four humours: blood, phlegm, yellow bile and black bile. A balance of these fluids resulted in health. In the case of cancer, an excess of black bile reportedly collected in various body sites (American Cancer Society 2004). In the Dark Ages little progress was made.

Cancer epidemiology

During the Renaissance, starting in the fifteenth century, scientists in Italy developed a greater understanding of the human body, mainly as a result of postmortem examinations and a clearer understanding of the organs of the body. In the seventeenth century, Bernardino Ramazzini, an Italian physician, noted the high incidence of breast cancer in nuns and suggested that it was in some way related to their celibate lifestyle. This launched cancer epidemiology, the study of the occurrence, distribution and control of the disease in the population. This was followed in the eighteenth century by the description of scrotal cancer in chimney sweeps by Sir Percival Pott, which led to many studies that identified a number of occupational carcinogens and then to public health measures to reduce cancer risk (Yarbro et al. 2000, American Cancer Society 2004).

Cancer surgery

Giovanni Morgagni laid the foundations of surgical oncology during his work with the pathology of cancer *post mortem* and John Hunter, a Scottish surgeon, applied this to practice (Yarbro et al. 2000). In the mid-nineteenth century, with the advent of anaesthesia, surgeons emerged who rapidly advanced surgical techniques for cancer: Theodor Bilroth in Germany, W. Sampson Handley in London and William Stewart Halsted in America. Their work led to cancer surgery designed to remove all of the tumour, as well as the regional lymph nodes, on the understanding that cancer was contained within anatomical compartments and metastasis spread via the lymph vessels. This thinking dominated cancer surgery for almost a century, until it was called into question by the work of twentieth century surgeons.

At the same time as Halsted and Handley, another surgeon, Stephen Paget, was researching metastatic spread and concluded that blood vessels, as well as the lymph, were involved and that the disproportionate spread of metastases to certain organs could not be the result of chance. Paget drew an analogy between metastases and seeds that were carried in all directions but could live and grow only on fertile soil; therefore cells from a tumour were able to grow only in certain organs – not just any organ where they came to rest. Paget's work contributed to a new understanding of cancer that still applies today (Yarbro et al. 2000, American Cancer Society 2004). The understanding of metastasis became a key element in the recognition of the limitations of cancer surgery. It allowed doctors to develop systemic treatments that were used before and after surgery to destroy cells that spread through the body, enabling the use of less mutilating surgery (American Cancer Society 2004).

Cancer treatments

In 1878 Thomas Beatson, a graduate of Edinburgh University, discovered that the breasts of rabbits stopped producing milk after he removed the ovaries, drawing the conclusion that one organ (the ovaries) has control over the secretion of another separate organ. Beatson tested this by the removal of ovaries in women with advanced breast cancer and found that it resulted in some improvement. He discovered the stimulating effect of oestrogen on breast cancer even before the hormone itself was discovered. Beatson's work provided the foundation for the modern use of hormone therapy in the treatment of breast cancer (Yarbro et al. 2000).

In 1896, Wilhelm Conrad Roentgen, a German physicist, discovered the X-ray, X being the algebraic symbol for an unknown quantity. Within 3 years, radiation was being used in the treatment of cancer. Unfortunately, radiation was recognized as a cancer-causing agent 7 years after its discovery, and a few years later a relationship with leukaemia was recognized (Yarbro et al. 2000). Today radiation is delivered with great precision to destroy tumours while preserving normal tissue (American Cancer Society 2004).

During World War II, naval personnel exposed to mustard gas as a result of military action were found to have severe bone marrow depression. In the studies that followed, a compound called nitrogen mustard was studied and found to have an effect on cancer of the lymph nodes. From this work, the development and use of chemotherapy drugs resulted in the successful treatment of many people with cancer. Cancers that can be cured with chemotherapy include lymphoma, acute childhood leukaemia, testicular cancer and Hodgkin's disease. Many other cancers can be controlled for long periods of time if not cured.

More recently, scientists' understanding of the biology of cancer cells has led to the development of biological agents that mimic natural signals used by the body to regulate growth. This cancer treatment, commonly referred to as biotherapy or immunotherapy, has proved effective for the treatment of several cancers.

Cancer in the twentieth century

James Watson and Francis Crick received the Nobel Prize for their work in the discovery of the exact structure of DNA, which enabled scientists to understand how genes work and how they could mutate. There was already an understanding that cancer could be caused by chemicals, radiation and viruses, and that sometimes cancer seemed to run in families. With the study of DNA it was discovered that damage to DNA by chemicals and radiation or the introduction of new DNA sequences by viruses led to the development of cancer. It therefore became possible to pinpoint the exact site of damage to a specific gene; it was also discovered that these damaged genes can be inherited.

Cancer biology

The normal cell and cell cycle

The body is made up of about 200 different types of cell. Each cell is a functional unit and arises from existing cells by a process of cell division. The cell is made up of three key parts: the plasma membrane, cytoplasm and nucleus.

Plasma membrane

This is the cell's outer surface which is made up of fats and proteins. The membrane allows substances to move in and out of the cell and restricts the movement of some substances. The function of the plasma membrane is determined by its protein make-up.

Cytoplasm

This is made up of all the cellular contents apart from the nucleus. There is a fluid portion, namely cytosol, within which are small organs termed 'organelles'; each organelle has a characteristic structure and function (Tortora and Grabowski 2004).

Cytosol

This is the fluid inside the cell; it makes up 55% of the cell's volume and is composed of water, solutes and particles. The cytosol is the site of many of the chemical reactions that allow cellular growth (Gabriel 2004, Tortora and Grabowski 2004).

Organelles

Each organelle is a functional unit where specific processes take place:

- Cytoskeleton: a network of protein filaments that maintains the shape and organization of the cell.
- Centrosome: made up of proteins important in cell division.
- Cilia and flagella: cilia are hair-like projections extending from the surface of the cell which propel fluids across the surface of cells. Cilia present in the cells of the respiratory tract sweep foreign particles trapped in mucus away from the lungs. Flagella are longer than cilia and can move entire cells; the only example in the human body is the tail of the sperm cell.
- Ribosomes: these are the sites of protein formation and they are made up of proteins and nucleic acids.
- Endoplasmic reticulum (ER): a network of folded membranes taking up half of the cytoplasm. It consists of rough ER and smooth ER. The rough ER is studded with ribosomes, and it processes and sorts proteins formed by the ribosomes. The smooth ER does not contain ribosomes and its function is the formation of fatty acids and steroids; it also plays a part in the inactivation of harmful substances including carcinogens.
- Golgi complex: made up of membranous sacs it stores packages and exports proteins from the rough ER to other parts of the cell.
- Lysosomes: made up of sacs containing 60 different digestive enzymes that break down the final products of digestion and allow them to be transported into the cytosol. Lysosomes also digest worn-out organelles (autophagy) and can destroy themselves (autolysis). Autolysis occurs in some medical conditions and also occurs after death when tissue deteriorates.
- Peroxisome and proteasome: peroxisomes detoxify harmful substances and proteasomes break down unneeded, faulty or damaged proteins.
- Mitochondria: these are the power house of the cell where energy is produced. Some cells contain thousands of mitochondria, but others just a

hundred, e.g. active cells such as the liver, kidneys and muscle have large numbers of mitochondria and use up lots of energy (Gabriel 2004, Tortora and Grabowski 2004).

Nucleus

This is a spherical or oval structure, usually the most prominent feature of the cell. Most cells have a nucleus with the exception of mature red blood cells; some cells, e.g. skeletal muscle cells, have several nuclei. The nucleus contains one or more spherical nucleoli that are clusters of protein, deoxyribonucleic acid (DNA) and ribonucleic acid (RNA), which engineers ribosomes.

Within the nucleus are most of the cell's hereditary units or genes, which control cellular structure and direct cellular activities. Genes are arranged in a single row on chromosomes. Human body cells have 46 chromosomes; 23 are inherited from each parent cell. The total genetic information carried in a cell is called its genome (Tortora and Grabowski 2004).

Gene action or protein synthesis

The main job of the cell is protein production or synthesis. The proteins determine the physical and chemical characteristics of the cell and in turn of the organism. The DNA contained in genes provides instructions for making proteins. The information in the DNA is copied to produce a specific molecule of RNA, which attaches to a ribosome where the information from the RNA is translated into a sequence of amino acids that goes on to form a new protein molecule.

DNA consists of repeating building blocks called nucleotides. Each nucleotide is made up of three parts: a nitrogenous base, deoxyribose and phosphate.

The nitrogenous bases consist of one of the following nucleic acids: adenine, guanine, thymine or cytosine. The DNA is made up of two strands, similar to a ladder, which twist around each other, giving it the double helical structure. The strands consist of alternating deoxyribose and phosphate groups, and the 'rungs' of the ladder contain the nitrogenous bases made up of one of the nucleic acids, the 'rungs' being formed when the nucleic acids from each strand join together in sequence: adenine always paired with thymine and cytosine with guanine. About 1000 rungs of DNA make up a gene, and humans have between 35 000 and 45 000 genes.

Any change that occurs in the sequence of the nucleotides (known as adenosine, or A, guanosine or B, thymidine or T and cytidine or C) of a gene is known as a mutation. Mutations can result in the death of a cell, cause cancer or produce genetic defects (Gabriel 2004, Tortora and Grabowski 2004).

Cell division

Cell division replaces damaged, diseased and worn-out cells. There are two different types of cell division:

1. Meiosis or reproductive cell division produces sperm and eggs, the cells needed to form the next generation of sexually reproducing organisms.
2. Mitosis or somatic cell division produces two identical cells after division in all other body cells (Gabriel 2004, Tortora and Grabowski 2004).

Mitosis

A cell divides into two identical cells by replication of the DNA sequence so that the same genetic material can be passed on to the newly formed cells. The cell cycle is the term used for the sequence of events occurring from the time a cell forms until it duplicates and divides (Gabriel 2004, Tortora and Grabowski 2004).

The cell cycle

- Interphase: a state of high activity during which the cell replicates its DNA and manufactures additional organelles in anticipation of cell division. As DNA replication starts the helical structure of the DNA partly uncoils and the rungs of the ladder containing the nucleic acids separate. The nucleic acids then pair up with the newly synthesized DNA. This uncoiling and pairing continues until each of the two original DNA strands is joined to the newly formed DNA strand. The original has become two identical DNA molecules.
- Mitotic phase: mitosis or division of the nucleus occurs followed by division of the cytoplasm into two cells. The duplicated chromosomes segregate, one set moving into each of two separate nuclei (Tortora and Grabowski 2004).

Each human cell has the same DNA content but only a small number of genes are expressed, giving each cell a distinct structure and function – termed 'differentiation'.

Carcinogenesis (cancer growth)

Carcinogenesis or cancer growth can be split into three stages:

1. Initiation: environmental, systemic or genetic changes to the gene.
2. Promotion: expression of mutant genetic information even after long periods of latency, sometimes by the initial promoter or carcinogen.
3. Progression: cells assume malignant behaviour, invade adjacent tissues and metastasize.

There are three main causes of cancer:

1. Environmental factors, diet, industrial pollution and viruses: studies of patterns of cancer around the world suggest that the key environmental factors related to cancer are smoking, diet, alcohol and sexual habits, and that some cancers may be avoidable if the environmental agent is removed.
2. Systemic factors, including the breakdown of the immune system.
3. Genetic factors that give rise to a degree of susceptibility for cancer.

Research suggests that cancer results from an interaction of factors at the cellular, genetic, immunological and environmental levels (Souhami and Tobias 1998, Yarbro et al. 2000, Gabriel 2004). Theories of tumour development suggest that cancer is an accumulation of mutations resulting from multiple events that act together.

Control of cell division is carefully maintained by opposing sets of genes, which promote and inhibit growth. Damage to genes is repaired by enzymes that are coded by DNA-repair genes. When damage cannot be repaired, the cell is destroyed. The number of times a cell is allowed to replicate is also controlled and limited. Growth-promoting genes are termed 'oncogenes' and growth inhibiting genes 'tumour suppressor genes'. The terminology used to describe growth regulation reflects the fact that the genes were initially thought to be cancer genes; normal cellular genes are often termed 'proto-oncogenes', adding to the confusion!

Carcinogenesis or cancer growth occurs when these genes are damaged to such an extent that normal control mechanisms for growth spiral out of control. For cancer to develop, oncogenes (growth-promoting genes) must be activated, tumour suppressor genes (growth-inhibiting genes) inactivated, DNA-repair genes inactivated and cell death blocked, and the biological clock turned off so that cells can become immortal (Souhami and Tobias 1998, Yarbro et al. 2000, Gabriel 2004). This process occurs with damage to the genome as a result of environmental, systemic and genetic factors. Oncogenes become mutated and are activated, and tumour suppressor genes and DNA-repair genes are mutated and become inactivated. It is common for mutated tumour suppressor genes or DNA-repair genes to be inherited, but inheritance needs to be from both parents for it to have an effect. Oncogenes are dominant genes and inheritance of a mutated gene is therefore necessary from only one parent for the effect to be shown.

Cancer may be thought of as a defect in the control of the cell cycle: tumour suppressor genes regulate checkpoints in the cell cycle, and if this does not occur growth is not controlled. It may also be thought of in terms of programmed cell death: mutated cells with defective DNA are induced to undergo programmed cell death or apoptosis. This process is defective in cancer cells (Souhami and Tobias 1998, Yarbro et al. 2000). Cancer can finally be thought of in terms of evolution and natural selection: the mutated gene eventually takes control until the host dies.

The effect on the cell

Altered cell growth

There is immortality, contact inhibition is lost (the property that stops normal cells growing when they come into contact with other cells), adhesion is lost (cells hold less firmly to each other), and there is loss of cell cycle control and programmed cell death. Cancer cells tend to be poorly differentiated, and in some cancer cells the tissue of origin cannot be confirmed.

Cytological

There is increased size and number of nucleoli, reflecting greater metabolic need and activity.

Changes in cell membrane

New surface antigens are exhibited.

Metastasis

Metastasis is the major cause of cancer death; in many cases metastatic spread occurs before the initial diagnosis of cancer.

Metastasis is the spread of tumour cells to a new site in the body via the bloodstream or lymph system (Gabriel 2004). To support tumour growth and movement, angiogenesis or formation of a blood supply occurs. Newly formed blood vessels provide nutrition and oxygen to the growing tumour, as well as being a potential travel route to other parts of the body. The degree of angiogenesis in the primary tumour is directly linked to metastatic spread and is the subject of research. Tumour cells also need to be motile (to move spontaneously without aid); again some research centres on anti-motile agents to reduce metastasis. Tumour cells have enzymes that allow surrounding tissues to be invaded and immunosuppressive factors that evade destruction by the immune system. Distribution of metastasis is not random and is probably related to tumour cell characteristics; tumour cells may lodge in the capillary beds of multiple organs, and certain microenvironments determine whether tumour growth is supported. Despite a lack of knowledge about the exact mechanisms of metastasis, research continues with a view to interrupting this process (Souhami and Tobias 1998, Yarbro et al. 2000, Morgan 2001, Gabriel 2004).

The classification and staging of cancer

Histology

This defines the tumour according to the tissue from which it arises:

- Carcinoma or epithelial tissue, e.g. the urinary tract, the colon, the respiratory tract
- Sarcoma or connective tissue, e.g. bone, muscle, blood
- Neural tissue, e.g. nerve cells.

Grading

This is a method of classification based on the histopathological characteristics of the tissue. One description of the microscopic appearance of cancer cells is the degree of differentiation or specialist function of the cell. All normal cells start as immature cells and when mature they carry out a specialist function, i.e. skin cells, bone cells or muscle cells. Normal cells that become cancerous lose their specialist function, and cancers that resemble the normal tissue of origin in appearance and function are well differentiated. Undifferentiated tumours show little or no resemblance to their tissue of origin and tend to be more aggressive. The grades are as follows:

- GX: grade cannot be assessed
- G1: well differentiated
- G2: moderately well differentiated
- G3: poorly differentiated
- G4: undifferentiated.

It is anticipated that a grade 1, well-differentiated tumour offers a good prognosis for the patient. Undifferentiated tumours show little or no resemblance to their tissue of origin and tend to be more aggressive. There are some problems with grading: several grades may exist within one tumour and the grade may vary over time (Souhami and Tobias 1998, Yarbro et al. 2000, Fawcett and Drew 2002).

Staging

Staging is used to establish the extent of disease at presentation. Staging is a clinical and histological tool and is one of the methods used to indicate prognosis and determine treatment options for solid tumours (Morgan 2001, Fawcett and Drew 2002). The TNM (tumour, node and metastases) system is one of several ways of staging cancers and is one of the most popular possibly as a result of its simplicity. T stands for primary tumour and the relevance of local invasion, N for lymph node spread and M for the presence of distant metastases (Souhami and Tobias 1998, Morgan 2001, Fawcett and Drew 2002) (Table 1.1).

Table 1.1 TNM staging

Stage	Size
T1	> 2cm in diameter
T2	2–5 cm in diameter
T3	> 5cm in diameter
T4	A tumour of any size with direct extension to chest wall or skin
N0	No palpable node involvement
N1	Mobile ipsilateral nodes
N2	Fixed ipsilateral nodes
N3	Supraclavicular or infraclavicular nodes or oedema of arms
M0	No distant metastases
M1	Distant metastases

Incidence and risk factors

Cancer is a major cause of illness in the UK, with more than 270 000 new cases diagnosed in the year 2000, 65% of these being diagnosed in people aged over 65. The main site-specific cancers are breast, lung, colorectal and prostate; together they make up over half of all new cases (Cancer Research UK 2004).

Breast cancer is the most common cancer in the UK, with over 40 000 cases per year; it is the most common female cancer and accounts for one in three of all female cancers. The second most common cancer in women is colorectal cancer with around 16 333 cases, followed by lung cancer with 15 200 cases (Cancer Research UK 2004).

In men the most common cancer is prostate cancer, making up 21% of all male cancers, closely followed by lung cancer at 18% and colorectal cancer at 14%.

The latest available mortality statistics indicate that, in 2002, 155 180 people were registered as dying from cancer. Cancer causes 26% of all deaths in the UK and 22% of those deaths are from lung cancer, with cigarette smoking identified as the single most important cause of preventable disease and premature death in the UK (Cancer Research UK 2004).

Cancer Research UK (2004) offers the following advice for reducing the risk for cancer.

Smoking

Smoking is the greatest avoidable risk factor for cancer, causing nine out of ten cases of lung cancer. Smoking is also a risk factor for cancer of the bladder, kidney, cervix, throat (pharynx and larynx), mouth, oesophagus, pancreas and stomach, and for some types of leukaemia. The three main components of cigarettes are nicotine, carbon monoxide and tar. Nicotine is not a carcinogen but is very addictive, carbon monoxide is a poisonous gas taken up by the bloodstream that impairs breathing, and tar is made up of various chemicals, many of which are known carcinogens. It is estimated that 70% of the tar in cigarettes is deposited in the lungs. Smoking is linked to socioeconomic status, manual workers being more likely to smoke than non-manual workers. The risk of getting lung cancer if you are a smoker is directly related to the number of cigarettes smoked: the higher the number, the higher the risk. This is also directly related to the length of time that the person has smoked. Risk of lung cancer is drastically reduced by stopping smoking; smokers who stop before the age of 35 have a life expectancy not significantly different from non-smokers, so the longer you do not smoke the more the risk is lowered.

Alcohol

Drinking too much alcohol increases the risk of mouth, throat and oesophageal cancer, and has been linked to breast cancer. Drinking and smoking together also have an effect on the risk for these cancers. People classed as alcoholics are at an increased risk from liver and bowel cancer. Government guidelines for drinking recommend three to four units per day for men and two to three units per day for women. One unit of alcohol equates to half a pint of beer or lager, a small glass of wine or a small fortified wine (port or sherry).

Diet

One-third of all cancers are related to diet; research suggests that dietary intake influences the risk of bowel, stomach, mouth, pharyngeal, oesophageal and pancreatic cancers, and is linked to breast, prostate, lung, cervical and bladder cancers. A healthy balanced diet should include fruit and vegetables, at least five portions per day. Research also suggests that eating fruit and vegetables protects against certain types of cancer. Measurement of dietary components and their relationship to cancer are the focus of long-term research. Dietary fibre found in cereals, vegetables and fruit protects the bowel from cancer by reducing constipation, a known risk factor for bowel cancer. Diets high in red and processed meat are linked to an increased risk for bowel cancer and are also linked to breast, lung, prostate and pancreatic cancers.

Obesity

Obesity is linked to some cancers, e.g. in women the risk of uterine cancer is higher. There is also a link to postmenopausal women and breast cancer possibly as a result of higher levels of circulating oestrogen (a known risk factor for breast cancer) linked to fat cells. Body mass index (BMI) (height in metres squared, divided by weight in kilograms) should be between 20 and 25, although this should not be looked at in isolation – it is only a rough guide.

Exercise

A combination of regular exercise, a healthy BMI and a healthy diet protects against a number of cancers. The recommended amount of exercise for a healthy lifestyle is 30 minutes of moderate exercise every day for 5 days a week. Moderate exercise includes brisk walking, swimming, cycling, vacuum cleaning, dancing, gardening and even pushing a pram. A combination of a healthy diet, healthy body weight and regular exercise has been shown to protect against a number of different cancers.

Safe sex

Some types of cancer have been linked to a virus transmitted through sexual intercourse. The human papillomavirus (HPV) has 70 different strains, some of which are more likely to cause cancer than others. The risk of cancer transmitted by HPV increases with many sexual partners, or by having unprotected sex. The use of condoms is advocated to reduce the risk.

Safety at work

The key risk factors for cancer in the workplace are asbestos, carcinogenic chemicals, and ultraviolet (UV) and ionizing radiation. Exposure to asbestos can also cause lung cancer (mesothelioma or cancer of the lining of the lungs), although there is a long delay between exposure to asbestos and disease development. Workers exposed to asbestos in the 1950s and 1960s, when regulations for the control of asbestos in the workplace were not in force, are only now showing signs of cancer development. Carcinogenic chemicals include: benzene, present in oil and gas and used in the petroleum industry; benzidine dyes, used in the textile industry; chromate pigments, used in the paint industry; and some herbicides and fertilizers. Carcinogenic chemicals are strictly controlled and all should carry hazard warnings by law. UV radiation, the harmful rays of the sun, increases the risk of skin cancer for people who work outdoors, unless sun protection cream and the covering up of exposed skin are encouraged. Ionizing radiation in high levels can cause cancers, in particular leukaemia. The nuclear industry, as well as the medical and dental professions, work with radiation sources that need adherence to strict health and safety guidelines. Ionizing radiation can be produced by X-ray machines or by gases such as radon, which are released naturally into the environment. It is estimated that 4% of all cancer deaths may be caused by exposure to a cancer-causing substance at work.

Sun and UV light

There are over 65 000 new cases of skin cancer reported every year in the UK, although the disease is almost totally preventable through methods of skin protection. Skin cancers are linked to prolonged exposure to the sun; UV radiation penetrates deep into the skin cells causing gene damage. People most at risk are those with a large number of moles or fair freckled skin, light coloured eyes and fair or red hair, particularly babies and children. People with dark skin that tans easily are less at risk. To protect skin from UV radiation: take care not to burn; avoid the midday sun; and cover up with loose clothing, a hat, sunglasses and suncream with a sun protection factor of at least 15, and avoid the use of sunbeds.

Family history

A small percentage of cancers (5–10%) are caused by faulty genes inherited from one parent. A familial history of cancer might be identified if there are several cases of the same type of cancer in one family, if cancers occur under the age of 50 or on the same side of the family, and if cancer types run together in families where there is a known link, i.e. breast and ovarian cancer.

In general it is important to know your own body and what is normal for you. Some body changes can be early warning signs of cancer. If action is swift there is a much better chance of successful treatment.

Conclusion

In the UK the lifetime risk of developing cancer is one in three with the risk rising significantly in people over the age of 65 (Cancer Research UK 2004). For health-care professionals working in this area, a clear understanding of the biology of cancer and its epidemiology and aetiology are necessary. This will help in caring for patients from prevention of cancer to its diagnosis and treatment.

References

American Cancer Society (2004) The History of Cancer: www.cancer.org
Cancer Research UK (2004) www.cancerresearchuk.org/aboutcancer/whatiscancer/version=2
Fawcett T, Drew A (2002) The classification, grading and staging of cancer development. Prof Nurse 17: 470–2.
Gabriel J (ed.) (2004) The Biology of Cancer. London: Whurr.
Morgan G (2001) Making sense of cancer. Nurs Stand 15(20): 49–53.
National Institutes for Health (2004) http://science.education.nih.gov/supplements/nih1/cancer/guide/understanding1.htm

Souhami R, Tobias J (1998) Cancer and its Management. Oxford: Blackwell Science.
Tortora G, Grabowski S (2004) Introduction to the Human Body: Essentials of anatomy and physiology, 6th edn. New York: John Wiley & Sons.
Yarbro CH, Frogge MH, Goodman M, Groenwald SL (eds) (2000) Cancer Nursing Principles and Practice, 5th edn. Boston, MA: Jones & Bartlett.

Chapter 2

Health promotion in cancer care

The number of deaths from cancer continues to fall; 155 000 people died from cancer in 2002 in the UK (Cancer Research UK 2004a). Although cancer mortality is falling, the incidence of cancer continues to rise, with 270 000 new cases registered in 2001 (Cancer Research UK 2004b). Four major types of cancer – breast, lung, colorectal and prostate – account for half of all cases diagnosed (Cancer Research UK 2004a). Much of the increase is likely to be the result of people living longer; however, lifestyle has an important part to play. The increase in incidence highlights the need to help prevent people developing cancer (Department of Health or DoH 2000).

> Better prevention, better detection of cancer and better treatment of cancer matter to us all.
>
> Department of Health (2000, p. 5)

This chapter looks at prevention strategies for the common cancers. It also focuses on screening in general terms, as well as discussing the national screening programmes relating to these cancers.

In defining health, the World Health Organisation's (WHO's) definition from its 1948 constitution is well known to professionals and lay people and defines health as a complete state of physical and mental well-being, not just an absence of disease (Sadler 2002). Sadler (2002) goes on to highlight the WHO's definition of health promotion as a process of enabling people to increase control over and improve their health.

The development of prevention strategies reinforces the view of health promotion as having a primarily preventive function in relation to cancer care; however, prevention is only one element of health promotion (Sadler 2002). Tannahill (2000) proposes a model of health promotion based on three overlapping spheres of activity:

1. Health education: enhancing health and well-being mainly through communication.
2. Prevention: risk reduction or avoidance, mainly through medical intervention, e.g. screening.
3. Health protection: safeguarding society's health mainly through legislative and fiscal policy.

The holistic nature of such definitions is to be embraced within cancer care; however, it is also noted that, in health care, such goals are often worked towards but not always realized (Sadler 2002). Over the last decade the expectations placed on nurses as health promoters have increased dramatically resulting partly from the major inequalities in health in the UK (DoH 2000, Whitehead 2001). *The NHS Cancer Plan* (DoH 2000) highlights the fact that unskilled workers are twice as likely to die from cancer than their professional counterparts. People from less affluent backgrounds are more likely to get some types of cancer and overall are more likely to die from it once they have been diagnosed. Lung cancer offers an example of the gulf between the different strata in society: in the early 1990s deaths from the disease among men were nearly five times higher among unskilled workers than among professional groups (DoH 2000). In the UK average fruit and vegetable consumption (known to protect against some cancers including bowel cancer) is approximately three portions a day; however, those in low-income groups eat fewer fruit and vegetables than those in high-income groups (DoH 2000). For many people a diet rich in fruit and vegetables is not an option, and the specific health benefits of fruit and vegetables in preventing cancer are not widely known, with many thinking that they are already eating enough (DoH 2000). Tannahill (2000) suggests that a multifaceted strategy is needed to address the needs of a multifaceted society, incorporating health education, prevention and protection.

Leavel and Clarke (1965) proposed a framework of primary, secondary and tertiary health promotion and this can be a useful for considering the different stages of a cancer journey.

Levels of health promotion

There are three levels of health promotion:

1. Primary: at the onset of the disease, predominately through education.
2. Secondary: prevention of progression of disease, e.g. screening for breast or prostate cancer.
3. Tertiary: intervention aimed at reduction of further disability or recurrence of disease when disease is already present, e.g. symptom management, rehabilitation and targeted patient education.

Prevention of cancer is a major aim of *The NHS Cancer Plan* (DoH 2000). As has been stated there are many causes of cancer, including genetic, environmental and lifestyle factors incorporating issues such as poverty and unemployment. For the most common forms of cancer, smoking and poor diet are by far the most important factors that need tackling from a health promotion point of view (DoH 2000).

Smoking

Smoking is the single greatest cause of preventable illness and early death in the UK. More than 120 000 people a year in the UK die from smoking and around 13 million adults smoke. More cigarettes are smoked per person in the UK than the European average and more deaths are caused by smoking than in other countries. Smoking costs the NHS up to £1.7 billion a year and passive smoking kills hundreds every year (DoH 1999). The White Paper *Smoking Kills* (DoH 1999) outlined three challenging targets:

1. To reduce smoking among children from 13% to 9% or less by the year 2010 with a fall to 11% by the year 2005.
2. To reduce adult smoking in all social classes so that the overall rate falls from 28% to 24% or less by the year 2010 with a fall to 20% by the year 2005.
3. To reduce the percentage of women who smoke during pregnancy from 23% to 15% by the year 2010 with a fall to 18% by the year 2005.

The government's tobacco strategy sets out a comprehensive plan of action and targets three groups. It seeks to reduce the number of those under the age of 16 years who smoke. It wants to help adults, especially disadvantaged individuals, to stop smoking and also to give special support to pregnant women. To achieve these targets the government believes that a range of steps will help prevent young people from starting to smoke and also help those who do to stop. Minimal tobacco advertising in shops and tough enforcement on under-age sales through the use of a proof-of-age card and strong rules on the siting of cigarette vending machines are some such steps (DoH 1999). Current debate is focused on the possibilities of banning cigarette smoking in public places. According to the Department of Health (1999) 70% of adults who smoke say that they want to quit. Some £60 million has been invested in new services to help people stop smoking, starting in the most deprived areas in England, which have been designated health action zones. General practitioners can refer people who want to stop smoking for specialist smoking cessation advice and nicotine replacement therapy is available on prescription (DoH 2000).

Other strategies in *Smoking Kills* (DoH 1999) include a major media campaign that aims to shift behaviour and reduce smoking. A new charter on smoking within the licensed trade and consultation on a new code of practice on smoking at work to protect the welfare of new smokers are being considered.

Diet

The NHS Cancer Plan (DoH 2000) identifies diet as the second most common cause of cancer after smoking, thought to be responsible for a third of all such deaths. Early studies have linked a high incidence of colorectal cancers in the west to the high fat and meat content of the western diet (Cancer Research Campaign 1998). High fat has also been linked to the development of breast cancer (Nicholson 1996).

Increasing the consumption of fruit and vegetables can significantly reduce the risk of many chronic diseases (WHO 1990, DoH 1994). It has been estimated that eating at least five portions of a variety of fruit and vegetables each day could reduce the risk of deaths from chronic diseases such as heart disease, stroke and cancer by up to 20% (DoH 2000). An increase in fruit and vegetable consumption is the second most important cancer prevention strategy after a reduction in smoking (DoH 2000). In 1998 the Department of Health Committee on Medical Aspects of Food Policy and Nutrition concluded that higher vegetable consumption would reduce the risk of colorectal cancer and gastric cancer and might reduce the risk of breast cancer. These cancers combined represent about 18% of the cancer burden in men and about 30% in women (DoH 1998). The advice to eat at least five portions or 400 g of a variety of fruit and vegetables each day is consistent with dietary recommendations around the world including those from the WHO (1984).

The National Fruit Scheme will make a free piece of fruit available to schoolchildren aged 4–6 each school day in pilot schemes in health action zones. This aims to increase fruit and vegetable consumption by raising awareness of the health benefits and improving access to fruit and vegetables through targeted action.

Other factors

Several other risk factors that can contribute to the development of cancer are highlighted within *The NHS Cancer Plan* (DoH 2000): obesity, physical activity, alcohol, sunlight and exposure to radon. Obesity can contribute to the risk from breast cancer and endometrial cancer; a diet low in fat can lower the risk and this is addressed within *The NHS Cancer Plan* (DoH 2000). Regular physical activity can lower the risk from some cancers such as colon cancer; *The NHS Cancer Plan* (DoH 2000) encourages physical activity promotion schemes, including the promotion of walking and cycling. Safe cycling routes have been implemented and advertised across the UK as well as walk to school and work schemes. Alcohol is implicated in 3% of cancers, notably cancers of the mouth and throat, and is the focus of the development of an alcohol misuse strategy. Sunlight is the main cause of skin cancer, which in line with other cancers continues on an upward trend (DoH 2000). Studies show that, although most people are aware of the risks from overexposure to the sun, few people take any precautions to protect themselves from the risk (DoH 2000). Society's association between a suntan and good health, perpetuated by the media, is a major determinant in health-promoting behaviour (Sadler 2002). Exposure to the radioactive gas radon increases the risk of lung cancer; the Department of Health is working closely with the Department of the Environment to investigate those areas of the country most affected (DoH 2000).

Screening

Screening is a public health service in which members of a defined population, who do not necessarily perceive that they are at risk of or are already affected by a disease or its complications, are asked a question or offered a test to identify those individuals who are more likely to be helped than harmed by further tests or treatment to reduce the risk of a disease or its complications (www.nationalscreeningcouncil.nhs.uk). Screening has important ethical implications because apparently healthy people are targeted. Screening has the potential to save lives or improve the quality of life through early diagnosis of serious conditions. Where screening is possible, it is an important method of detecting abnormalities at an early stage, affording treatment when the cancer has the greatest chance of cure or, in some cases, before it even develops (DoH 2000). It is not a foolproof process; in any screening programme there are false-positive results – those wrongly reported as having the condition – and false-negative results – those wrongly reported as not having the condition.

The principles underlying decisions about screening, advocated by Wilson and Jungen (1968, cited in James 2002), are still applied today:

- The condition sought should be an important health one.
- There should be an accepted treatment for patients with recognized disease.
- Facilities for diagnosis and treatment should be available.

- There should be a recognized latent or early symptomatic stage.
- There should be a suitable test or examination.
- The test should be acceptable to the population.
- The natural history of the disease, from latent phase to declared disease, should be adequately understood.
- There should be an agreed policy about whom to treat as patients.
- The cost of case finding (including diagnosis and treatment of patients diagnosed) should be economically balanced in relation to possible expenditure on medical care as a whole.

People invited to participate in screening programmes need to have some understanding of the potential benefit and harm in doing so and be sufficiently empowered to make an informed choice about whether or not they wish to proceed. Information therefore needs to be honest, comprehensive and understandable (DoH 2000).

Breast cancer

Over 41 000 women are diagnosed with breast cancer every year, making it the most common cancer in the UK (Cancer Research UK 2000, page 3270). The NHS Breast Screening Programme (NHSBSP) screens women from the age of 50 to 70 by taking a radiograph (mammogram) of the breast, the aim being early detection to reduce mortality. Data from Swedish clinical trials have shown an overall reduction in breast cancer mortality of 29% during 12 years of follow-up in women aged 50 who were invited for screening (Blamey et al. 2000). However, some researchers would argue that the contribution of screening to decreasing mortality rates is impossible to evaluate with any accuracy, and point out the fact that improvements in survival rates predate the inception of the NHSBSP in 1990. Other researchers insist that it has saved thousands of lives and will go on doing so, in particular related to quality improvements in the screening process and staff expertise (DoH 2000, Carlisle 2002).

Women aged 50–70 are invited for screening; invitations are taken from a GP's lists, and it should be noted that this excludes a proportion of women not registered with a GP. Those women over the age of 70 are also entitled to screening every 3 years on request, the balance between effective screening and radiation risk being a key determinant in the 70+ age group (DoH 2000).

At the inception of the breast-screening programme in the UK, one view of the breast was taken at mammography; research evidence incorporated into guidelines published in *The NHS Cancer Plan* (DoH 2000) suggests that two views can increase detection rates by 43%. This research is being implemented across the country to ensure that each woman screened is offered the best screening possible.

Cervical cancer

In 2000 there were 2424 new registrations of invasive cervical cancer in England (Cancer Research UK 2000). Although the incidence rates are slightly below the European average, the mortality rates are slightly above (Cancer Research UK 2003a). Cervical cancer is the eleventh most common cause of cancer deaths in women in the UK, accounting for around 2% of all female cancers (Cancer Research UK 2003b)

For the first time ever, death rates from cervical cancer have fallen below 1000 in England: in 2002, 927 deaths were registered (Cancer Research UK 2003a). Mortality rates in 2000 were 60% lower than they were 30 years earlier; cervical screening now saves about 1300 lives per year (Sasieni and Adams 2003).

Cervical screening began in Britain in the mid-1960s. By the mid-1980s, although many women were having regular smear tests, there was concern that those at greatest risk were not being tested and that those women who had positive results were not being followed up and treated effectively. The NHS Cervical Screening Programme was set up in 1988 when the Department of Health instructed all health authorities to introduce computerized call and recall systems. The programme screens almost 4 million women in England each year (DoH 2001–2002).

Although cervical screening cannot be 100% effective, screening programmes have been shown to reduce the incidence of cancer in a population of women. A single screen at the age of 40 years reduces the cumulative incidence of cervical cancer by 20% (Miller 1992), whereas annual screening between the ages of 20 and 64 reduces the cumulative incidence of cervical cancer by 93.3% (Hakama et al. 1986)

Future developments in cervical screening

Liquid-based cytology

Research suggests that the use of liquid-based cytology could provide significant and important benefits, namely reducing the number of false-negative test results as well as the number of unsatisfactory specimens. In addition, it may decrease the time needed for examination of specimens by cytologists (www.cancerscreening.nhs.uk). The National Institute for Clinical Excellence (NICE) undertook evaluation of the technique and has recommended its use. The date of implementation is yet to be announced (www.nice.org.uk).

Human papilloma virus

There are over 70 different types of this virus which are given numbers to distinguish them. Some types of human papilloma virus (HPV) are linked to cervical cancer, primarily numbers 16–18 (www.cancerresearch.uk.org). High-risk HPV types have been found to be present in close to 100% of all cervical cancers, and research has indicated that women with a mild or borderline smear result who have no evidence of high-risk HPV are very unlikely to develop cervical cancer (www.cancerscreening.nhs.uk). HPV testing has been proposed as a means of distinguishing women with a high risk of developing cervical cancer from those with a low risk. It is argued that a test for the HPV has the potential to become the main screening tool for preventing cervical cancer. A recent study involving 11 000 British women aged 30–60 found that the test for HPV detected 97% of significant cervical abnormalities compared with 76% for the smear (Cuzick and Szrewski 1995). The Medical Research Council has funded the Trial of Management of Borderline and Other Low-grade Abnormal smears (TOMBOLA). Recruitment started in December 1999 and the trial will include 10 000 women between the ages of 20 and 59 years.

Two new leaflets have been launched to give women clear, honest and balanced information about the benefits of cervical screening, meeting the commitment in *The NHS Cancer Plan* (DoH 2000). There are plans for an audio version and an English Braille version of the leaflets. The leaflets have also been translated into five languages so that women can make a genuinely informed choice about whether or not to accept their invitation for screening. There are plans to translate the leaflet into a further 12 languages.

Colorectal screening

Bowel cancer is the third most common cancer in the UK, affecting 34 000 people annually. Around 13 000 people will die from the disease every year. It often develops from small growths called polyps, some of which are precancerous adenomas that can eventually progress to full-blown cancer. This process takes about 10 years, during which time bowel cancer can be prevented by removing the benign growths. A major new study by Cancer Research UK scientists found that screening looks capable of cutting incidence and mortality from the disease by 40% in the target age range. The study involved 170 000 people and tested the ability of a technique called flexible sigmoidoscopy to detect and treat bowel cancer. It found that screening is feasible, safe and effective, with the potential to prevent around 5000 cases of the disease each year in the UK (Ransohoff 2002). The National Screening Committee (NSC) found that population screening of people over the age of 50 years for the presence of occult (non-visible) blood in the faeces can reduce the mortality rate for bowel cancer (Hardcastle et al. 1996, Kronborg and Fenger, 1996). Two pilot sites for screening were set up in 1999 in Coventry and Warwickshire in England, and Tayside, Fife and Grampian in Scotland. For a 2-year period men and women aged between 50 and 69 years of age, who were registered with a participating GP, were offered a faecal occult blood test (FOBT) to screen for bowel cancer. The pilot ended in 2002. The evaluation report has been submitted to the NSC and the Department of Health in England and Scotland, and a national bowel cancer screening programme based on the report and other relevant research will be developed. A second round of screening is now under way.

Prostate cancer

Every year over 27 000 men are diagnosed with prostate cancer in England and Wales and over 9000 men die from the disease (Cancer Research UK 2003b). Screening for prostate cancer is a controversial issue. There are no known primary prevention measures that men can take to minimize the risk of developing prostate cancer (DoH 2000). Screening methods available can show false positives, which can lead to unnecessary investigation or even treatment for some men, and be detrimental to their health (Austoker 1994). Prostate-specific antigen (PSA) is a glycoprotein secreted by the prostate and its level rises as a man ages (James 2002). A raised PSA might indicate the presence of prostate cancer, but there is not enough evidence to advocate a screening programme. In screening for prostate cancer, healthy men are invited to have a blood test that is able to detect a cancer that has not caused symptoms; early detection has not been shown to increase survival. For some men slow growing tumours, if left untreated, might never cause problems and in fact some never present clinically (James 2002). For many men disease progression is slow and they can die with prostate cancer rather than because of it (James 2002).

The government, in its NHS cancer programme, confirms that there is not enough evidence to recommend a national screening programme; however, trials are currently under way with the National Cancer Institute and European Cancer Programme to compare the screened and unscreened populations and subsequent survival. These studies involve 74 000 and 50 000 men; results will be available in 2010 (Templeton 2003).

Ovarian cancer

Ovarian cancer is the fourth most common cause of cancer deaths in women in the UK, resulting in 4500 deaths each year (DoH 2000). Symptoms of ovarian cancer do not become evident until the disease is advanced and, although there are tests available to screen for ovarian cancer (transvaginal ultrasonography and a blood test for a cancer antigen CA-125), research suggests that there is insufficient evidence to promote screening. According to *The NHS Cancer Plan* (DoH 2000), the government will consider screening when research demonstrates that it is cost-effective and appropriate.

Lung cancer

There is at present no screening technique that is sensitive enough to be used for mass screening; however, low-dose spiral computed tomography has been identified as a method to identify asymptomatic individuals at high risk. Research is currently ongoing (DoH 2000).

Behaviour change

Central to targeting health promotion at all levels is the need for individuals to change their behaviour. Becker (1974) devised the health belief model as a means of bringing about and understanding change. This model is based on a 'cost–benefit exercise': any action will be based on the payback that the individual receives. It is argued that individuals need to have certain beliefs to undertake certain behaviours (Becker 1974). The model can be useful in helping health professionals understand and predict health behaviours, and can help us to understand why some individuals find it difficult to change behaviour, e.g. stopping smoking, despite having knowledge of the consequences. Critics of the model argue that all the factors are given equal weighting and the actions of an individual can appear oversimplified. Preventive measures will not necessarily prevent a cancer occurring. Examples of the health belief model are shown in Table 2.1.

Table 2.1 Examples of the health belief model

Factors needed to predict a course of action	Adverse effects of sun exposure
Incentive to change	Sunburn during a holiday
Must feel threatened by current behaviour	A suspicious mole
Change must be perceived to be beneficial	Is it better to have a pale skin after a holiday than to increase the risk of developing skin cancer?
Must feel competent to carry out change	Is sun protection affordable?
Must be a cue to bring about this change	Leaflet as part of a campaign, article in a magazine, contact with a health-care professional

Conclusion

The implementation of *The NHS Cancer Plan* (DoH 2000) has raised public and professional awareness of health promotion and cancer care. The plan specifically targets the issues of cancer prevention, largely through investment in smoking cessation campaigns and encouraging people to eat more fruit and vegetables. Health promotion is a means of maintaining well-being on receiving a diagnosis of cancer and during treatment, as well as before any cancer has been detected. Health promotion in cancer care is often seen as the preserve of nurses working at a primary care level. Nurses have a responsibility for maximizing health potential at all stages of the disease continuum. Patients are gaining a greater level of knowledge about their health or illness and, according to Webb (1994), patient education is in fact commonly referred to as 'tertiary health promotion'. Patient education is being integrated into all aspects of care and should be concerned with communicating with patients, identifying need, exploring myths and misconceptions, and wherever possible offering truly individualized care. The nurse working with cancer patients in any health-care setting has a role to play in health promotion.

References

Austoker J (1994) Screening for ovarian, prostatic and testicular cancers. BMJ 309: 315–20.
Becker M (1974) The Health Belief Model and Personal Human Behaviour. Thorofare, NJ: Slack.
Blamey RW, Wilson ARM, Patnick J (2000) Screening for Breast Cancer. In: Dixon JM (ed.), ABC of Breast Diseases, 2nd edn. London: BMJ Books, pp. 33–7.
Cancer Research Campaign (1998) UK Incidence Fact Sheet no. 11. London: CRC.
Cancer Research UK (2000) National Statistics, Cancer Registrations in England 2000: www.cancerreasearch.uk
Cancer Research UK (2003a) Health Statistics Quarterly. National Statistics. London: Cancer Research UK.
Cancer Research UK (2003b) National Statistics, Cancer Registrations in England 2003: www.cancerresearch.uk.
Cancer Research UK (2004a) Incidence UK: www.cancerresearchuk.org/statistics.
Cancer Research UK (2004b) Mortality UK: www.cancerresearchuk.org/statistics.
Carlisle D (2002) Cancer: the big picture. Nurs Times 98(35): 22–4.
Cuzick J, Szrewski A (1995) Human papillomavirus testing in primary cervical screening. Lancet 345: 1533–7.
Department of Health (1994) Nutritional Aspects of Cardiovascular Disease. London: HMSO.
Department of Health (1998) Our Healthier Nation: A contract for health. London: DoH.
Department of Health (1999) Smoking Kills. London: DoH.
Department of Health (2000) The NHS Cancer Plan: A plan for investment, a plan for reform. London: DoH.
Department of Health (2001–2002) Statistical Bulletin 2001–02 Cervical Screening Programme: www.cancerscreening.nhs.uk.

Hakama M, Miller AB, Day NG (1986) Screening for Cancer of the Uterine Cervix. Lyon: IARC.
Hardcastle JD, Chamberlain JO, Robinson MHE (1996) Randomised controlled trial of faecal occult blood screening for colorectal cancer. Lancet 348: 1472–7.
James N (2002) Prostate cancer screening: the pros and cons. Cancer Nurs Pract 1(3): 22–5.
Kronborg O, Fenger C (1996) Randomised study of screening for colorectal cancer with faecal occult blood test. Lancer 348: 1467.
Leavel H, Clarke H (1965) Preventive Medicine for the Doctor in his Community. New York: McGraw Hill.
Miller AB (1992) Cervical Cancer Screening Programmes. Geneva: WHO.
Nicholson A (1996) Diet and the prevention and treatment of breast cancer. Alternative Therapies 2; 32–38; 20.
Ransohoff DF (2002) Lessons from the UK sigmoidoscopy screening trial. Lancet 359: 1266–8.
Sadler C (2002) Health promotion in cancer care. Cancer Nurs Pract 1(3): 26–31.
Sasieni P, Adams J (2003) Benefits of cervical screening at different ages: evidence from the UK audit of screening histories. Br J Cancer 89: 888.
Tannahill A (2000) Working to a Healthier Nation. Edinburgh: Health Education Board for Scotland.
Templeton H (2003) The management of prostate cancer. Nurs Stand 17(21): 45–53.
Webb P (ed.) (1994) Health Promotion and Patient Education. A professional guide. London: Chapman & Hall.
Whitehead D (2001) A social cognitive model for health education/health promotion practice. J Adv Nurs 36: 417–25.
Wilson J, Jungen G (1968) Principles and Practice of Screening for Disease. Public Health Paper no. 34. Cited in James (2002), p. 24.
World Health Organisation (1948) Constitution for Health. Geneva: WHO.
World Health Organisation (1984) Health Promotion: A discussion document of concepts and principles. Geneva: WHO.
World Health Organisation (1990) Diet, Nutrition and the Prevention of Chronic Disease. Geneva: WHO.

Chapter 3

Colorectal cancer

In the UK, colorectal cancer is the second most common cancer in the women and the third most common in men (Cancer Research UK 2003). The disease can occur at any age but is most common in elderly people and rare in those aged under 40 (Cancer Research UK 2003). The incidence of colorectal cancer is increasing, attributed in part to a high-fat, low-fibre diet and limited exercise (Scottish Intercollegiate Guidelines Network or SIGN 1997). As with other cancers, although the incidence is increasing – 1 in 25 will develop the disease – mortality is decreasing partly as a result of early detection and different treatment options and lifestyle changes (Campbell and Borwell 1999, Borwell 2002, Knowles 2002). As mentioned above, colorectal cancer is uncommon in the under-40 age group, incidence increasing with age and affecting both genders equally up to the age of 60, after which the incidence is slightly higher in men (Behrand 2000, Borwell 2002).

Cancer patients in England often have poorer survival prospects than in other European countries resulting partly from advanced disease at first presentation (Department of Health or DoH 2000). Colorectal cancer typically has a late presentation and is therefore more advanced at diagnosis. *The NHS Cancer Plan* (DoH 2000) has a remit to detect cancers earlier by raising public awareness. Screening and early detection are also important methods for reducing morbidity and mortality, as well as improvements in treatment (Ellis and Sadler 2000).

Anatomy and physiology

The gastrointestinal tract is made up of the mouth, pharynx, oesophagus, stomach and intestines. The primary function of the tract is to provide cells with nutrients and water. The large intestine is divided into the caecum, ascending colon, transverse colon, descending colon, rectum and anal canal (Figure 3.1). The small intestine opens into the large intestine at the caecum in the right lower abdominal quadrant; the ileocaecal valve allows the contents of the intestine to pass in one direction only (Walsh

1999, Ellis and Sadler 2000). The appendix, a blind-ended tube, is attached to the caecum and is a frequent site of inflammation and infection. The large intestine ascends the right side of the abdominal cavity from the caecum as the ascending colon, and flexes at the undersurface of the liver to form the transverse colon. The descending colon passes down the left side of the abdomen and becomes known as the sigmoid colon because it takes an S-shaped course through the pelvis (Walsh 1999). The rectum is a continuation of the sigmoid colon. It is about 15–17 cm long and contains vertical folds, each of which contains an artery and vein; the veins may become varicose, forming haemorrhoids. The terminal portion of the gastrointestinal tract opens on to the surface of the body at the anus. The opening between the rectum and the anal canal is controlled by the internal anal sphincter, and the anus is controlled by the external anal sphincter (Walsh 1999).

Figure 3.1 Anatomy of the intestines

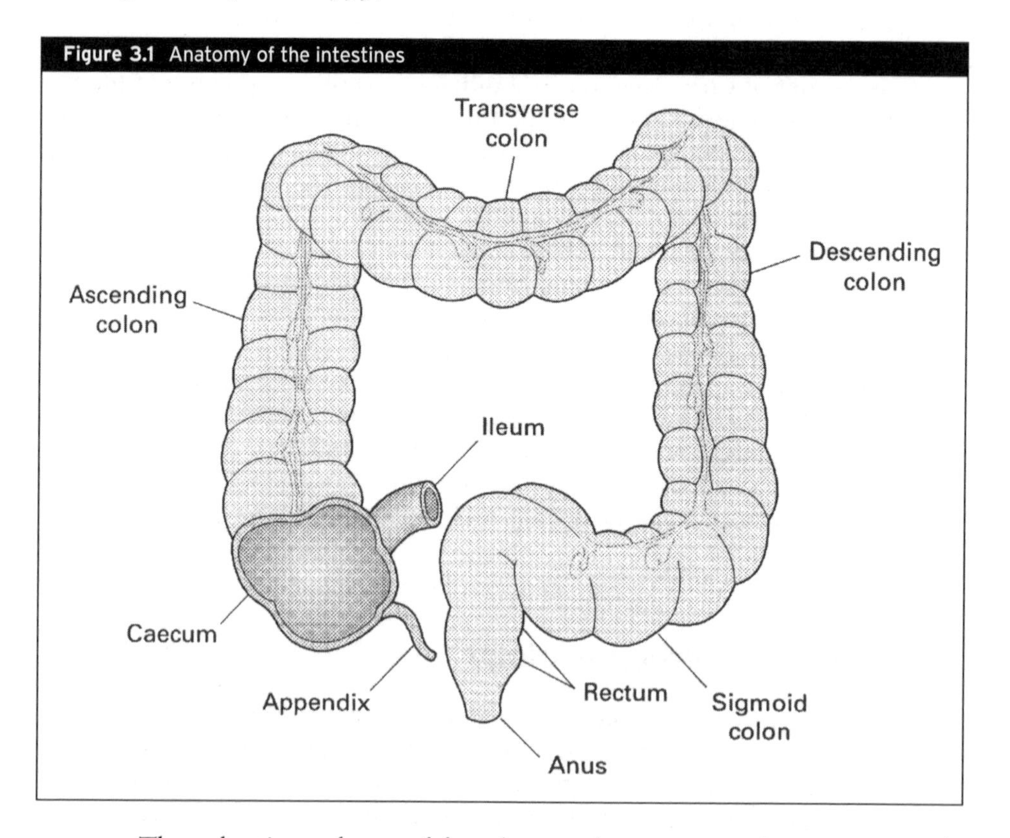

The colon is made up of four layers: the mucosa, submucosa, muscle and serosa. The mucosa and submucosa are divided by the muscle layer (Ellis and Sadler 2000). Contraction of the muscular tissue in the large intestine (peristalsis) mixes the contents as well as propelling them towards the rectum three to four times a day. Water is added to the content of the gastrointestinal tract as part of the digestive process. However, in the colon much of this water is reabsorbed, changing the consistency of the content to a soft solid mass referred to as faeces (Walsh 1999).

Defecation is the expulsion of faeces from the rectum, which normally remains empty until just before this process. Faeces entering the rectum cause local distension and pressure causes sensory nerve impulses to initiate reflex impulses to the internal anal sphincter with the result that it relaxes (Walsh 1999).

Faecal matter consists of mucus, gastric secretions, water, unabsorbed food residue and micro-organisms. If faecal matter is moved too rapidly through the large intestine, less water is absorbed and the stool is unformed and liquid. If movement and elimination are delayed, an excessive amount of water is absorbed and the faecal matter becomes hard and dry (Walsh 1999).

Irritation of the large intestine can result in secretion of mucus (more than is usual to lubricate faecal matter and facilitate movement), as well as water and electrolytes, in an effort to dilute the irritant; this can cause faecal matter to remain in liquid format (diarrhoea) resulting in dehydration and electrolyte imbalance (Walsh 1999).

If the faecal matter is hard and dry and defecation is delayed, the result is termed 'constipation'. This can have several causes but is frequently associated with a lack of fibre (resulting in less residue) in the diet and a sedentary lifestyle, as well as disease.

Risk factors

Many risk factors are associated with the development of colorectal cancer, including age, ethnicity, genetic predisposition, pre-existing bowel disease, history of other cancers and lifestyle.

Diet is thought to be one of the key risk factors associated with colorectal cancer; studies consistently demonstrate an association between lack of fruit and vegetable consumption and cancer (Knowles 2002). Diets high in fibre reduce the transit time of the faecal bulk in the colon, so potential carcinogens have less contact time with the bowel mucosa (de Snoo 2002). Lifestyle and environmental factors are significant when discussing risk. Recent work by Giovannucci (2001) has shown an elevated risk of colorectal cancer from cigarette smoking, although previous evidence remains inconclusive. Obesity in men, high alcohol consumption and reduced physical activity and mobility are all key factors (Cummings and Bingham 1998, Kiningham 1998, Knowles 2002).

The incidence for developing colorectal cancer increases slightly at 40 years and then dramatically at age 50, doubling each decade thereafter. In general younger people have a worse outcome; this is generally thought to be a result of the late presentation of disease in younger people (Behrand 2000). Incidence rates for colorectal cancer are highest in North America, northern and western Europe, New Zealand and Australia (European Oncology Nursing Society or EONS 2000, Knowles 2002). As with some other cancers, studies of migrants suggest that their risk of developing cancer changes from that of their own country to that of the host country very quickly, with environmental factors playing a key role (Cohen and Winawer 1995).

Family history

Family history plays a significant part in colorectal cancer, the risk being five times greater than that of the general population (SIGN 1997). Being at risk is defined as having two or more relatives with colorectal cancer, one of whom is under 55 years old, or one relative with colorectal cancer under the age of 45 years (Knowles 2002). There are specific genetic predispositions to colorectal cancer, including hereditary non-polyposis coli (HNPCC), a gene mutation characterized by at least three relatives with confirmed colorectal cancer, at least one being a first-degree relative, and two consecutive generations being affected with diagnosis under the age of 50 (Knowles 2002). HNPCC accounts for 5% of all new colorectal cancers (Summerton 1999). Familial adenomatous polyposis (FAP) is also caused by a gene mutation; it is characterized by the development of large adenomatous polyps in the colon and rectum, leading to the development of colorectal cancer. Individuals at risk should be offered a colonoscopy every 2–3 years and yearly sigmoidoscopy can be considered. Individuals with FAP can be offered proctocolectomy in which the anus, rectum and colon are removed and an ileostomy performed, or a total colectomy with lifelong check-ups of the residual rectum (Knowles 2002). FAP accounts for 1% of all new colorectal cancers (Summerton 1999).

Other high-risk factors include ulcerative colitis, when diagnosed under the age of 25 and with entire colon involvement for more than 7 years, and previous history of colon cancer and, in women, genital cancer (Cancer Research Campaign 1999).

Prevention

If colorectal cancer is detected early before the lymph nodes are involved, the 5-year survival rate can be as high as 70–80%. If spread has occurred to the regional lymph nodes and beyond, the 5-year survival rate is 25–30% (Rees and Williams 1995).

The food that we eat directly influences the risk of bowel cancer, which is predominantly associated with high-fat, red meat and low-fibre diets that are characteristic of a western lifestyle. Evidence suggests that a diet rich in vegetables, fruit, fibre, reduced fat and red meat reduces the risk of disease.

Screening

The aim of a screening programme is to identify asymptomatic disease and provide or have available treatments for those people whose disease is detected early (Borwell 2002). Screening can involve invasive procedures and can be costly. The introduction of a national screening programme should fulfil certain criteria: the disease should be an important health problem; there should be a recognizable early stage and a treatment available; treatment at an early stage should be more beneficial than later treatment; there should be a suitable screening test available; the test should be acceptable to the population, and reasonably simple and safe; and the test must be sufficiently sensitive and specific to give a high degree of accuracy. Sensitivity is the ability of a test to diagnose a condition correctly each time that it is used; specificity is the ability of a test not to diagnose someone as wrongly having the condition.

Faecal occult blood testing (FOBT) is under investigation as a screening method for the detection of colorectal cancer – stools are checked for blood that cannot be seen by the eye. A pilot study has been started in two sites in England and three in Scotland, and the results will underpin any decision to set up a national screening programme (Knowles 2002). FOBT remains controversial as a result of the nature of the testing; some people do not find it acceptable and sensitivity and specificity remain poor, yielding false positives as a result of ingestion of raw vegetables, horseradish, rare meat, iron supplements and aspirin (Behrand 2000, de Snoo 2002).

The disease

The route and presentation of symptoms vary as does the site. About 40% of cancers occur in the ascending, transverse and descending colon (Figure 3.2), with 25% in the sigmoid colon and the remaining 35% in the rectum (Borwell 2002). Presenting symptoms associated with right-sided tumours include: anaemia, weight loss, abdominal pain, an abdominal mass and a change in bowel habit. Left-sided tumours present with: abdominal cramping, and changed bowel habit with or without the passage of mucus and/or blood. Rectal tumours present with: passage of bright red blood mixed in the stool, and a feeling of unsatisfied defecation accompanied by persistent ineffectual spasms (Knowles 2002). Intestinal obstruction can also occur anywhere in the bowel and be linked to other conditions such as inflammatory bowel disease, irritable bowel syndrome and haemorrhoids. The main symptom leading to the detection of colorectal cancer is the change in bowel habit: constipation, diarrhoea and/or rectal bleeding (Knowles 2002). Some common presenting features are associated with metastatic spread of the disease rather than those related to the primary tumour and include: anorexia, fatigue, jaundice, bone pain, incontinence, intestinal obstruction or perforation.

Figure 3.2 Main sites of colorectal cancer

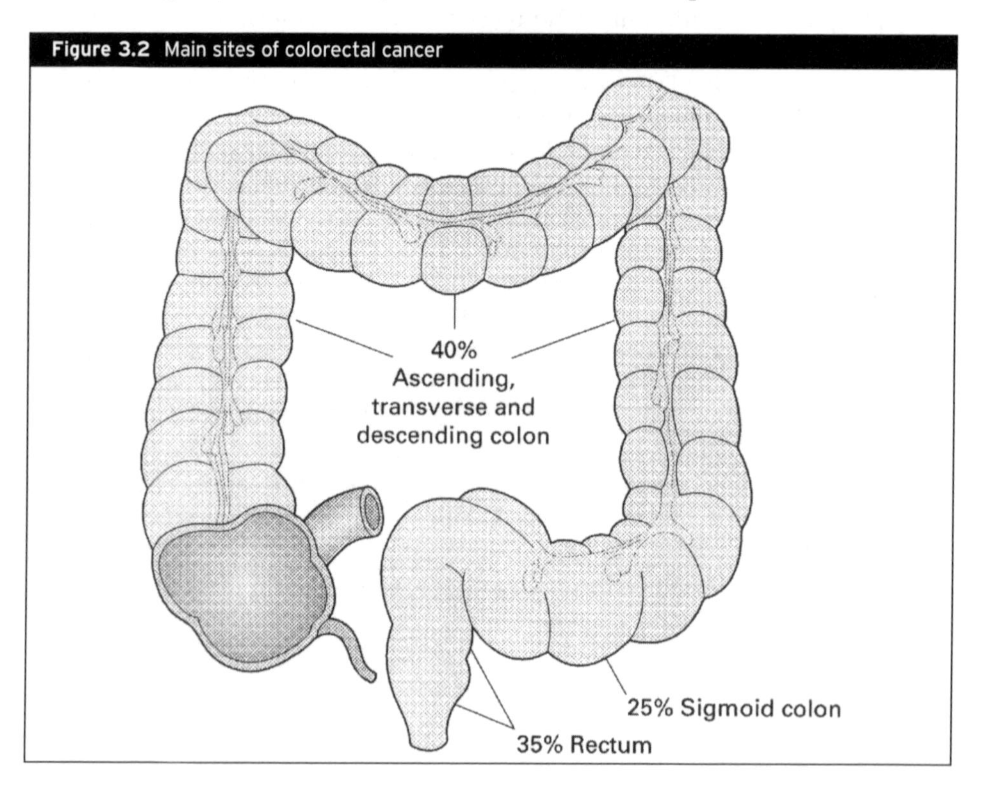

At diagnosis, 37% of colorectal cancers are localized, 37% have spread regionally to surrounding tissue, organs and lymph glands, and 19% have distant metastases (Knowles 2002). Dukes' classification of colorectal cancer stages the disease for prognostic indicators (de Snoo 2002):

- Dukes' A: invasion of the mucosa (innermost muscle layer of the bowel wall) – 95% 5-year survival rate.
- Dukes' B: penetration of mucosa into the serosa – 80% 5-year survival rate.
- Dukes' C: spread to lymph nodes – 50% 5-year survival rate.
- Dukes' D: metastatic disease – 5% 5-year survival rate.

There is evidence to suggest that there are significant delays from the onset of symptoms to treatment. Delays can be on the part of the patient or the GP, or within the hospital after referral (Summerton 1999). *The NHS Cancer Plan* (DoH 2000) highlights these issues and makes suggestions to decrease the time from onset to treatment. Health promotion regarding colorectal cancer is aimed at the prospective patient, clearer guidelines for referral for GPs and targets for waiting times once referred to hospital.

Diagnosis

Diagnosis involves completing a detailed patient history with clinical procedures to determine the site of the cancer, extent of local spread and distant metastases (Borwell 2002, Knowles 2002). Investigations include the following (Borwell 2002, de Snoo 2002, Knowles 2002):

- Digital rectal examination: a gloved finger is inserted into the rectum to feel any abnormalities; this test is easy to complete and is relatively pain free but only identifies 10% of colorectal cancers.
- Rigid or flexible sigmoidoscopy: a thin hollow tube with a light on the end is inserted into the rectum. The tube is connected to a video camera and can visualize the rectum and lower part of the colon. This test can visualize polyps when they are small but may miss cancerous polyps in the upper part of the colon.
- Double-contrast barium enema: an enema is given to make the colon visible by radiology; any abnormalities should show up.
- Colonoscopy: with the patient sedated, a thin flexible tube connected to a video camera is placed into the rectum and can examine the entire colon with biopsy for histological confirmation or to remove small cancers.
- Computed tomography (CT) to determine extent of the primary cancer and any metastatic spread.

- Magnetic resonance imaging (MRI) to determine local and metastatic spread.
- Endoanal ultrasonography to outline the layers of the rectal wall and detect lymph node involvement.
- Liver ultrasonography to detect metastatic disease.
- Chest radiograph to determine metastatic disease.
- Blood tests can also be used to determine disease present in the liver.

Treatment

Surgery

Conventional surgical management of colorectal cancer results in an overall 5-year survival rate of only 40%, so treatment includes adjuvant radiotherapy and chemotherapy after surgical resection (Information and Statistical Division or ISD 2000).

Planned or elective surgery usually involves a wide excision of normal bowel proximal and distal to the tumour, removing supporting tissue and lymph nodes, and is dependent on the anatomical site of the tumour.

Types of surgery

- For tumours of the colon and upper rectum, it is usually possible to join together the ends of the bowel where the cancer has been removed. This is referred to as an anastomosis (Figure 3.3).
- Occasionally a stoma is required; in some cases this is temporary to minimize leakage and encourage healing (Borwell 2002).
- Anterior resection is a sphincter-saving operation performed on the rectum. Two types of anterior resection are performed: high and low.
- Low anterior resection for tumours in the mid to lower third of the rectum is performed, usually with total mesorectal excision. This is used increasingly to reduce the incidence of local recurrence. The lower the tumour, the more rectum has to be removed, with significant consequences for the patient in relation to bowel frequency and continence. The coloanal pouch was introduced to improve the functional results of the lower anterior resection: an artificial rectum is formed, using a loop of colon joined to the anal canal.
- High anterior resections are used for tumours in the upper third of the rectum, leaving a short length of rectum to assist with bowel function. For those patients with tumours in the lower part of the rectum, an abdominoperineal resection may be necessary resulting in a permanent colostomy, although it is possible to reconstruct the rectum in tumours situated more than 5 cm from the anal verge (Figure 3.4).

Figure 3.3 Left hemicolectomy and anastomosis

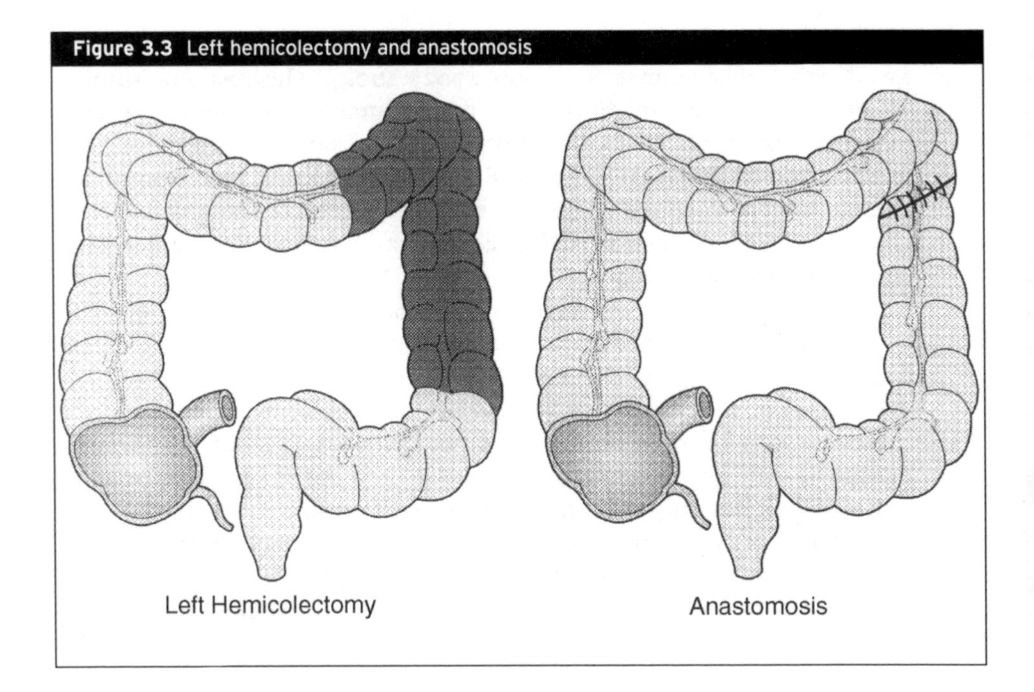

Figure 3.4 Abdominoperineal resection and colostomy

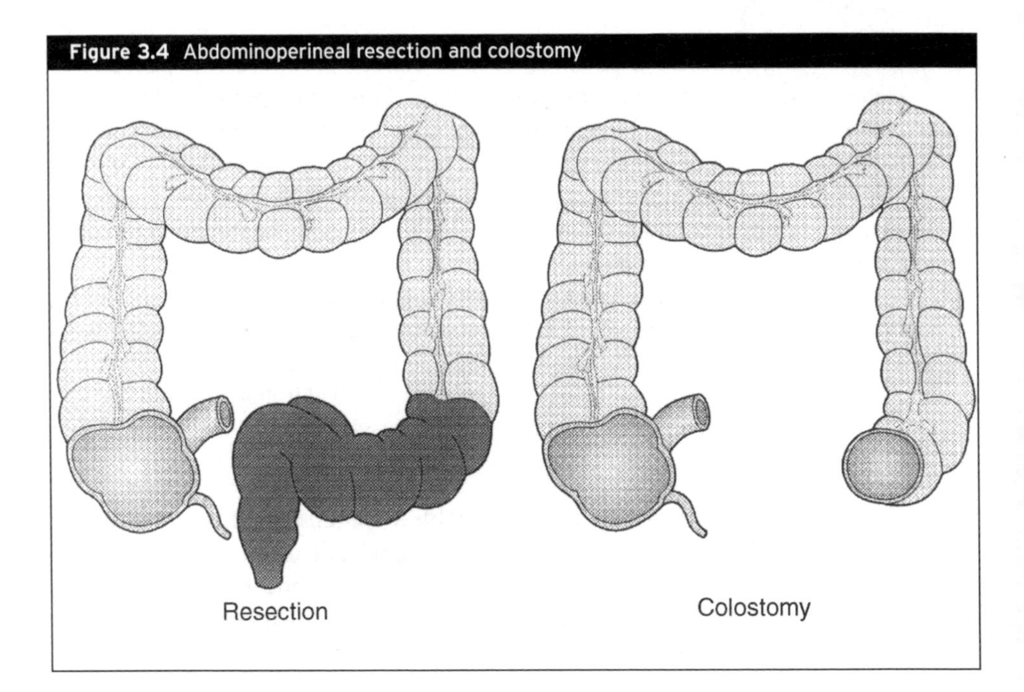

The surgical emphasis is moving towards sphincter-saving techniques that avoid permanent stomas (de Snoo 2002, 2004). The goals of surgical resection include complete removal of the tumour, disease-free surgical margins, dissection of local lymph nodes, a patent anastomosis and preservation of anorectal function (Eckhauser and Knoll 1997). Some colorectal surgery requires resections that may damage the pelvic nerves involved in sexual function. Other side effects may include faecal leakage and frequency (Borwell 2002).

Emergency surgery is sometimes necessary for an intestinal obstruction, perforation or excessive bleeding. Most obstructions occur in the descending colon where the lumen is narrow and faecal content solid. If the disease is widespread, or if tumour removal is impossible, surgical bypass or stoma formation is carried out. Surgical resection for metastatic disease can be carried out on solitary tumours in the liver or lung; however, this has only a limited cure (Borwell 2002).

Surgery, possibly with a stoma, has significant psychological and social consequences. Information about treatment options, side effects and prognosis is of particular significance and when holistically focused can help facilitate adaptation (Borwell 2002).

Radiotherapy

Radiotherapy can be used in colorectal cancer preoperatively, to downstage tumours in preparation for surgery. This gives patients with large tumours more surgical options and a greater chance of cure. Radiotherapy for local recurrence has been shown to improve local control of symptoms but not survival. Radiotherapy is also used palliatively to control disease, manage symptoms and improve quality of life (Nevidjon and Sowers 2000, Knowles 2002, Bulmer and Duthie 2004).

Radiotherapy is also associated with significant side effects, including fatigue, diarrhoea, sore skin and wound infections (Nevidjon and Sowers 2000, Knowles 2002).

Chemotherapy

Colorectal cancer is nearly always curable with surgery if detected in the early stages, but as has been stated more than half of all cases in the UK are diagnosed only after the cancer has spread beyond the bowel. A key priority in cancer research is to develop effective treatments for advanced disease (Cancer Research UK 2003).

Research studies suggest that the benefits of chemotherapy in colorectal cancer advocate that it be used in the main for Dukes' stage C colorectal cancer. Colorectal cancers that extend through the bowel wall or involve local lymph nodes tend to recur with distant metastases, using adjuvant chemotherapy alongside surgery has failed to demonstrate any significant advantage (Nevidjon and Sowers 2000). For some patients with advanced disease, the use of chemotherapy is essentially palliative, to reduce tumour load; however, several research studies are under way (Knowles 2002, Cancer Research UK 2003, Bulmer and Duthie 2004).

The side effects associated with chemotherapy include diarrhoea, nausea, fatigue, infection and altered taste (Knowles 2002).

Psychosocial effects

The psychological effects of cancer relate to a sense of loss, loss of health, opportunities, choice and control. These effects, as well as the uncertainty about the future, can lead to anxiety and depression (Grosser 2003).

Research has shown that, even after curative surgery for colorectal cancer, patients' quality of life can be poor. Patients who require stoma formation experience more problems, particularly in relation to body image and sexuality. Psychological effects of stoma surgery can be greater than the physical effects, the change in body image resulting in mourning for the lost body part, with surgery being viewed as an assault on body intactness. Concerns may also include fear of pain, mortality, anger, distress and disbelief (Black 2004).

Faecal incontinence and increased frequency of defecation are common in patients after low anterior resections and can continue for up to 2 years after surgery. Men can experience impotence and ejaculatory difficulties, whereas women might develop urinary problems including incontinence and dysuria (Camilleri-Brennan and Steele 1998). Many health professionals still fail to address sexuality in the clinical setting, focusing more on treatment outcomes and side effects (Horden 2000).

Social support is associated with better adjustment and decreased emotional distress and helps adaptation to a future of uncertainty. Nurses play an important role in informal support; support groups can also be an effective means of enabling adjustment (Lugton 1997).

The role of the nurse

The NHS Cancer Plan (DoH 2000) promotes patient-centred care, highlighting the need for patients to receive the treatment that they need when they need it. It also emphasizes the importance of communication between health-care professionals and between health-care professionals and patients to promote high-quality care and patient empowerment. Issues that patients highlight as being important are: being treated with humanity, dignity and respect; good communication; clear information; the best possible symptom control; and psychological support when necessary (DoH 2000).

Interdisciplinary team working and integrated care pathways can ensure a consistent and equitable approach to planning and managing care (Knowles 2002).

The role of the stoma specialist is widely acknowledged in terms of optimal functioning and support (Camilleri-Brennan and Steele 1998, Bulmer and Duthie 2004). Key issues for nurses include: the assessment of physical and psychological needs; information giving about the disease, its treatment, management of side effects, lifestyle changes and available support services; the planning of appropriate care with regard to treatment and side effects; the coordination of care to ensure an integrated seamless service; ongoing holistic assessment and monitoring; and excellent communication with the patient and other disciplines (Knowles 2002, Bulmer and Duthie 2004).

Conclusion

In the UK alone, there are 18 500 new cases of colorectal cancer in men and 16 000 new cases in women each year. The disease can occur at any age but is most common in the elderly and rare in the under-40 age group (Cancer Research UK 2003). If colorectal cancer is detected early before lymph nodes are involved, the 5-year survival rate can be as high as 70–80%. If spread has occurred to the regional lymph nodes and beyond, the 5-year survival is 25–30% (Rees and Williams 1995). Early detection is key to successful treatment and the Department of Health has in place initiatives to identify those at most risk, as well as promoting health education related to those factors known to contribute to the disease, e.g. diet.

Research is ongoing in key areas to investigate methods of screening, and improve treatment and care, as well as improving survival (DoH 2000, National Institute for Clinical Effectiveness or NICE 2004). Supportive care is essential if those affected by colorectal cancer are to be empowered to make treatment decisions along the cancer pathway and to have a good quality of life as they live with cancer.

References

Behrand S (2000) Colon cancer. In: Nevidjon B, Sowers K (eds), A Nurse's Guide to Cancer Care. Philadelphia, PA: Lippincott, pp. 83–134.

Black P (2004) Psychological, sexual and cultural issues for patients with a stoma. Br J Nurs 13: 692–7.

Borwell B (2002) Bowel cancer in the older person. Cancer Nurs Pract 1(4): 32–8.

Bulmer M, Duthie G (2004) Cancer of the lower gastrointestinal tract. In: Porock D, Palmer D (eds), Cancer of the Gastrointestinal Tract: A handbook for nurse practitioners. London: Whurr.

Camilleri-Brennan J, Steele R (1998) Quality of life after treatment for rectal cancer. Br J Surg 85: 1036–43.

Campbell T, Borwell B (1999) Colorectal cancer, Part 4: Specialist nurse roles. Prof Nurse 15: 197–200.

Cancer Research Campaign (1999) The Facts: Common Cancers: www.crc.org/cancer/Aboutcan_common.3html.

Cancer Research UK (2003) Briefsheet: Bowel cancer. Cancer Research UK.

Cohen A, Winawer S (1995) Cancer of the Colon and Rectum and Anus. St Louis, MO: McGraw-Hill.

Cummings J, Bingham S (1998) Diet and the prevention of cancer. BMJ 12: 1636–40.

de Snoo L (2002) Colorectal cancer. Cancer Nurs Pract 1(10): 32–8.

de Snoo L (2004) Anterior resection syndrome – the long term effects of surgery for rectal cancer. Cancer Nurs Pract 3(6): 23–7.

Department of Health (2000) The NHS Cancer Plan: A plan for investment, a plan for reform. London: HMSO.

Eckhauser FE, Knoll JA (1997) Surgery for primary and metastatic colorectal cancer. Gastroenterol Clin N Am 26 : 103–27.

Ellis C, Sadler D (2000) Colorectal cancer. In: Yarbro C, Frogge M, Goodman M, Groenwald S (eds), Cancer Nursing: Principles and practice, 5th edn. London: Jones & Bartlett.

European Oncology Nursing Society (2000) Colorectal Cancer. Brussels: EONS.

Giovannucci E (2001) An updated review of the epidemiological evidence that cigarette smoking increases risk of colorectal cancer. Cancer Epidemiol Biomarkers Prev 10: 725–31.

Grosser L (2003) The special needs of younger women. Cancer Nurs Pract 2(1): 13–14.

Horden A (2000) Intimacy and sexuality for the woman with breast cancer. Cancer Nurs 23: 230–6.

Information and Statistical Division (2000) Trends in Cancer Survival in Scotland 1971–1995. Edinburgh: ISD.

Kiningham R (1998) Physical activity and the primary prevention of cancer. Primary Care: Clinics in Office Practice 25: 515–36.

Knowles G (2002) The management of colorectal cancer. Nurs Stand 16(17): 47–52.

Lugton J (1997) The nature of social support as experienced by women treated for breast cancer. J Adv Nurs 25: 1184–91.

National Institute for Clinical Effectiveness (2004) Improving Supportive and Palliative Care for Adults with Cancer. London: NICE.

Nevidjon BM, Sowers KW (2000) A Nurse's Guide to Cancer Care. Philadelphia, PA: Lippincott.

Rees P, Williams D (1995) Principles of Clinical Medicine. London: Edward Arnold.

Scottish Intercollegiate Guidelines Network (1997) Management of Colorectal Cancer. Edinburgh: SIGN
Summerton N (1999) Diagnosing Cancer in Primary Care. Oxford: Radcliffe Medical Press
Walsh M (ed.) (1999) Watson's Clinical Nursing and Related Sciences. London: Baillière Tindall/RCN.

Chapter 4

Breast cancer

Over 41 000 women are diagnosed with breast cancer every year in the UK. It is the most common cancer in the UK and the most common cancer in women (Cancer Research UK 2004). For women, the lifetime risk of developing breast cancer is one in nine. With 1 million new cases in the world each year, breast cancer makes up 18% of all female cancers (McPherson et al. 2000). Most cases of breast cancer occur in postmenopausal women, but over 8000 women in the UK under the age of 50 are diagnosed each year as well as 300 men (Cancer Research UK 2004).

The incidence of breast cancer has increased over the past 30 years for a variety of reasons, including: better screening methods, better statistical records, and women living longer and being exposed to carcinogens; however, the mortality rate is decreasing, reflecting the benefits of early detection and screening, and improvements in treatment (Chapman and Goodman 2000, Nystrom et al. 2000).

It is well documented that early presentation of breast cancer improves outcome (Hermon and Beral 1995). It is also a remit of *The NHS Cancer Plan* (Department of Health or DoH 2000) to detect cancers earlier by raising public awareness and, although more women do consult earlier with breast cancer than other cancers, there is evidence to show that women in general are still not breast aware (Bailey 2000).

Breast anatomy and physiology

Breast development begins during weeks 7–12 of embryonic development. A ridge, known as the 'milk line', extends from the base of the upper limb to the base of the lower limb. From weeks 13 to 20 the epithelial bud branches to form the 15–20 major ducts found in the adult breast. Mature or cyclical development of the breast occurs in the female with the onset of puberty and an increase in oestrogen secretion. The adult female breasts lie on each side of the chest, extending into the axilla via a pyramid-shaped axillary tail. The nipple extends about 5–10 mm above the level of the areolar skin. The areolar has a number of openings:

large glands called Montgomery's glands which lubricate the areolar skin during suckling. The breast consists of lobes; each lobe is drained by a ductal system that opens into the nipple via a milk duct (Figure 4.1). Within the lobe there are up to 40 lobules, each 2–3 mm in diameter. About 48% of the breast tissue is made up of fat. The blood supply is from the axillary and mammary artery and drainage is from the intercostal and axillary veins. Lymph drainage from the breast is via the regional lymph nodes, most of which lie in the axilla. The axillary nodes can be divided into three groups in relation to the muscles of the chest wall: levels 1, 2 and 3. There are on average 20 nodes in the axilla, 13 at level 1, 5 at level 2 and 2 at level 3; lymph drainage passes from level 1 to 2 and then on to 3 (Bundred et al. 2000). Most benign conditions and almost all breast cancers arise within the terminal duct lobular unit.

Figure 4.1 Anatomy of the breast

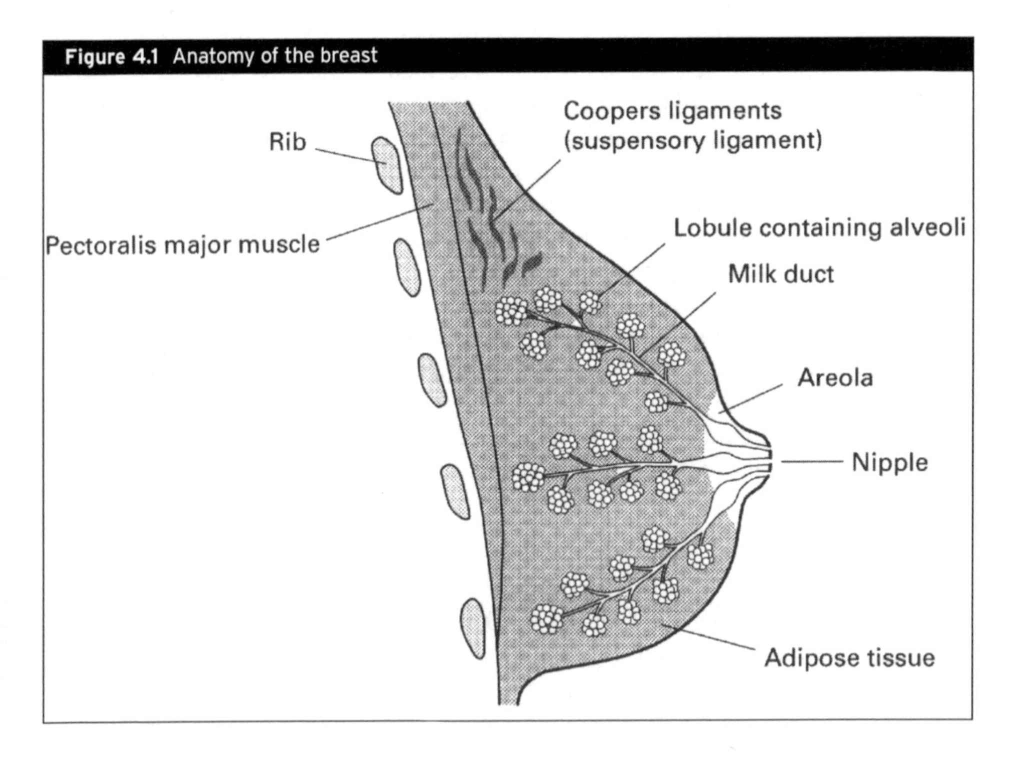

After the breast has developed, it undergoes changes related to the menstrual cycle and pregnancy. This is termed 'involution' and begins some time after the age of 30 or after pregnancy, breast stroma being replaced with fat so that the breasts become droopy (Dixon and Mansell 2000).

Risk factors

According to epidemiological factors related to breast cancer, every woman is randomly at risk of developing it at some time in her life; however, a number of risk factors can influence a woman's probability of developing the disease:

- Age remains the greatest risk factor, with most breast cancers occurring in the postmenopausal age group.
- There is evidence to suggest that hormones, in particular oestrogen, are related to the risk factors for breast cancer (McPherson et al. 2000).
- Women who start menstruating early, before the age of 11, are at increased risk.
- Those who have a late menopause, after the age of 55, are at increased risk (McPherson et al. 2000).
- The age of the woman at first pregnancy is thought to be significant; the highest-risk group are those who have their first child after the age of 35. Pregnancy has been reported to exert a deterrent effect on the development of breast cancer as a result of changes in hormone status. Lactation and breast-feeding have historical significance as protective mechanisms against breast cancer development, but this theory is controversial and thought to be related to pregnancy rather than breast-feeding alone (Chapman and Goodman 2000).
- Oral contraceptives and hormone replacement treatment (HRT) are also significant. There is a small risk associated with the oral contraceptive pill while the woman is taking it and for 10 years after cessation. Women who begin use before the age of 20 are at higher risk than women who start at an older age. There is a small risk associated with the use of HRT and for the first 1–4 years after stopping taking it (McPherson et al. 2000).
- Family history plays a significant part in breast cancer development; between 5% and 10% of breast cancers in western countries are the result of genetic predisposition; this can be passed on through either sex and does not always lead to the development of a breast cancer (McPherson et al. 2000). It is not known how many breast cancer genes there may be. There are almost certainly unidentified genes that increase the risk of breast cancer by a moderate degree. Two genes have been identified – *BRCA*-1 and *BRCA*-2 – and account for a large proportion of very-high-risk families (McPherson et al. 2000). Families affected by these mutations show an excess of ovarian, colon, prostate and other cancers. Women who develop bilateral breast cancer or breast cancer and another cancer, and women who get the disease at an early age, are most likely to be carrying a genetic mutation (McPherson et al. 2000). Most cancers caused by a genetic mutation will occur before the

age of 65. A woman's risk is increased by two or more times if she has a first-degree relative who developed the disease before the age of 50, i.e. a mother, sister or daughter. The younger the relative when the disease presented, the greater the risk. The risk increases by between four and six times if two first-degree relatives develop the disease (McPherson et al. 2000).

- Previous benign disease generally offers a slight increase in risk, e.g. cysts and fibroadenomas; however, in women with atypical epithelial hyperplasia (where the cells become atypical) the risk is four to five times higher than usual (McPherson et al. 2000).
- The incidence of breast cancer in western countries is five times that of countries in the Far East. Studies of migrants from Japan to Hawaii show that the incidence of breast cancer in the migrant assumes that of the host country within one to two generations, indicating that environmental factors are of greater importance than genetic factors.

The following lifestyle factors have some significance: there is thought to be a link between dietary fat intake and breast cancer and obesity is associated with an increased risk in postmenopausal women. Prolonged exposure to radiation is also associated with an increased risk of breast cancer (McPherson et al. 2000).

Family history

Women at high risk from breast cancer may be at high risk of other cancers and careful management is required (McPherson et al. 2000). Many breast units have family history clinics providing the genetic counselling and psychological support that women need. Many of these clinics incorporate nurse-led clinics with advanced nurse practitioners working very closely with women and their families (Page et al. 2000, Vogel 2003). Managing women at high risk includes: encouraging regular screening, prevention and performing bilateral subcutaneous mastectomies (Page et al. 2000). Current recommendations for screening advocate women being screened by mammography 5–10 years younger than the age of the youngest relative to have developed the disease, although there is no evidence that regular screening in the under-50 age group reduces mortality (Page et al. 2000). Breast cancer prevention trials using tamoxifen (an anti-oestrogen) found that the drug halved the risk of breast cancer development. Bilateral subcutaneous mastectomy has been shown to reduce breast cancer in women with a family history by about 90% (Page et al. 2000).

Prevention

There is a general lack of information about the cause of breast cancer; however, there are a certain number of risk factors, some of which are more significant than others. Research regarding prevention and early detection is critically important in the reduction of mortality, but 70% of women presenting with breast cancer have no identifiable risk factors (Chapman and Goodman 2000). According to Miller et al. (2000), the 5-year survival rate for a localized breast cancer is 84%, with regional spread 71% and distant metastases only 18%. In the UK, many women present with advanced disease at first presentation (DoH 2000).

Screening for breast cancer

Screening for breast cancer can encompass breast awareness, clinical breast examination and mammography. In the UK women are encouraged to be breast aware from the age of 18, when most female breasts have undergone mature development. Women need to be encouraged to be breast aware, knowing what is normal and what changes to look for:

- Lump in breast or axilla
- Area of thickening
- Dimpling or puckering of skin
- Alteration in appearance of nipple or breast
- Change in skin colour
- Discharge from nipple
- Discomfort in breast.

The use of breast clinical examination as a detection measure has not been proved and it is not used in the UK as a screening measure (Blamey et al. 2000).

The NHS Breast Screening Programme (NHSBSP 1998) screens women from the age of 50 to 70, the aim being early detection to reduce mortality (see Chapter 2).

The disease

Breast cancers occur in the epithelial cells that line the terminal duct lobular unit, part of the milk duct. Cancer cells that remain within the basement membrane are *in situ* or non-invasive, e.g. ductal carcinoma *in situ* (DCIS). An invasive breast cancer is one in which there is spread outside the basement membrane of the ducts and lobules into the surrounding tissue (Sainsbury et al. 2000). Some breast cancers have specific features, and are called a special type; the rest are no special type. Some breast cancers of a special type have a better prognosis than those of no special type. Cancers of no special type are graded by the degree of differentiation (how much they resemble the original cell). Low-grade tumours are well differentiated; high-grade tumours do not resemble the original cell and represent a more aggressive type of disease. Local lymphatic and vascular spread are also prognostic indicators, signalling an aggressive form of cancer.

The involvement of axillary lymph nodes with cancer has long been recognized as a key feature in prognostic assessment. Seventy per cent of patients with negative nodes survive for 10 years; this worsens as the number of positive nodes increases, with recurrence seen in 75% of patients with many positive nodes (Chapman and Goodman 2000).

Hormone receptor status is also useful in determining prognostic and treatment information. Normal breast tissue has hormone receptors that respond specifically to the stimulatory effects of oestrogen and progesterone. Most breast cancers retain oestrogen receptors and in these cancers oestrogen will retain control over the cancer cells. It is therefore useful to know the oestrogen receptor status of the cancer, in order to predict which patients will respond to hormone therapy. Cancers that lack hormone receptors will not respond to hormone therapy (Chapman and Goodman 2000).

Male breast cancer

Male breast cancer accounts for less than 1% of all breast cancers. The anatomical structures of the male breast are the same as those of the female breast. It is the hormonal stimulation present in the female breast, but absent in the male, that accounts for the developmental differences. Breast cancer in both sexes is similar in terms of risk factors, natural history and response to treatment. However, the presence of Klinefelter's syndrome (hormonal imbalance and gynaecomastia) increases the risk (Chapman and Goodman 2000).

Diagnosis

Diagnosis of breast cancer is made using the 'triple test':

(1) mammography
(2)clinical breast examination
(3)needle biopsy.

The triple test is successful in diagnosing the majority of palpable lesions. Needle biopsy is either a 'fine needle aspiration' for cytology or 'core biopsy' for histology. For screen-detected impalpable lesions, image-guided needle biopsy is necessary; this can be either mammographically or ultrasonically guided. In some cases a wire localization biopsy is necessary: a wire is placed next to the lesion in the breast under image guidance and an area around the wire excised. A preoperative definitive diagnosis for palpable lesions should be achieved in 95% of cases; the minimum standard for non-palpable lesions in the NHSBSP is 70% (Blamey et al. 2000). Multidisciplinary assessment is available to decide on appropriate management. The role of the nurse is very important within the diagnostic period when the woman may still be quite shocked, particularly if, as one of the screening population, she was a 'well woman' just a few days previously. The support afforded at this time can reduce distress in the pre-treatment period and also enhance the process of recovery and adjustment (Cimprich 1999).

Treatment

Surgery

Treatment for breast cancer consists of a combination of local treatments for local disease and systemic treatments for metastatic disease (secondary spread). For local disease the aim is breast conservation therapy or mastectomy and radiotherapy. Breast conservation therapy consists of excision of the tumour with a 1-cm margin of normal tissue; taking further tissue is a wide local excision or a quadrantectomy. Completeness of the excision is the key factor because invasive or *in situ* disease at the resection margins will increase the local recurrence rate. About one-third of breast cancers are not suitable for breast conservation and mastectomy is performed. Mastectomy involves removing the breast tissue with some underlying skin, leaving the chest wall muscles intact. Most patients treated by mastectomy are suitable for some form of breast reconstruction, which should ideally be performed at the same time as initial surgery (Chapman and Goodman 2000, Sainsbury et al. 2000). Complications after surgery include seroma formation (a collection of fluid under mastectomy flaps after drain removal) and flap necrosis (tissue death). The seroma can be easily aspirated and if necessary necrotic skin excised from the flaps. Limitation in mobility, including shoulder dysfunction and upper extremity weakness, can also be a problem; exercises to maintain mobility can start after 24 hours.

The presence or absence of involved axillary lymph nodes is the best predictor of breast cancer survival and it is used to make treatment decisions (Bundred et al. 2000). The number of nodes involved as well as the level of nodal involvement are significant. Some centres sample the axilla, looking to dissect four nodes, and find that this provides valuable information about the presence or absence of cancer. Other centres find the dissection of only four nodes difficult and follow the assumption that the probability of a false-negative result will decrease with the number of nodes sampled. Removal of all nodes at levels 1, 2 and 3 provides more accurate assessment of the number and level of nodal involvement (Bundred et al. 2000). Sentinel node biopsy is currently being researched as an alternative to extensive axillary surgery. The sentinel node is the first node in the lymphatic basin that receives primary lymph flow. The histological characteristic of the sentinel node is thought to predict the histological characteristics of the remaining lymph nodes in the axilla. The research involves injecting a radioactive substance into the area around the cancer, which later drains into the axilla. The axilla is then explored during breast surgery and the sentinel node identified and removed. If the sentinel node is positive, an axillary clearance can be undertaken. If the sentinel node is negative, the rest of the axilla is likely to be negative in 92–95% of cases and the patient can be spared an axillary dissection (Chapman and Goodman 2000). Several complications are associated with axillary dissection. Nerve damage may occur during surgery, causing numbness and paraesthesia down the upper inner aspect of the arm. Seroma formation can be a problem followed by wound infection in axillary procedures. Reductions in arm movement can occur and some patients require intensive physiotherapy. Axillary dissection can lead in some cases to lymphoedema (Bundred et al. 2000).

Intraductal carcinoma (or DCIS) rarely carries a risk of axillary node involvement. Options for treatment include mastectomy, wide excision followed by radiotherapy or wide excision alone. Invasive cancers develop in about 20% of patients within 10 years when excisional biopsy alone is selected as definitive treatment (Chapman and Goodman 2000).

It is important to note that most women who have not had immediate breast reconstruction after mastectomy will want some form of external breast prosthesis, although this is not always the case (Keeton and McAloon 2002). The fitting of a temporary breast prosthesis should be offered to all women before leaving the ward after surgery.

Radiotherapy

Studies have shown that all patients should receive radiotherapy to the breast after wide local excision or quadrantectomy. After mastectomy radiotherapy should be considered for patients at high risk of local recurrence, patients with muscle involvement and patients in whom there is axillary node involvement (Sainsbury et al. 2000). Modern machinery and treatments mean that the risk of complications from radiotherapy is minimal; some local reaction may be seen, and this can include mild erythema, dry desquamation or moist desquamation, when the integrity of the skin is lost and therefore predisposed to infection (Carroll 1998). If dermatological effects are present, the patient will need advice and support over skin care and dressings. Radiotherapy to the axilla can also contribute to lymphoedema.

Radiotherapy treatments are generally delivered daily over a 3- to 5-week period; supportive care at this time from nurses and radiographers cannot be overemphasized. In the aftermath of a cancer diagnosis and then surgery, daily visits can cause fatigue in the patient and also the family.

Chemotherapy

More than 50% of women with operable breast cancer who receive local treatment alone (surgery and radiotherapy) will die from metastatic disease; this points to the fact that in those women micrometastases were present at the time of initial presentation (Smith and deBoer 2000). The only way to improve survival is to administer systemic treatment either before (neoadjuvant) or after (adjuvant) surgery. The use of chemotherapeutic agents has been shown in clinical trials to improve survival. Combinations of chemotherapeutic agents have been shown to be more effective than single agents and the greatest benefit has been seen in women aged under 50. Common side effects of chemotherapy include hair loss, fatigue, lethargy, nausea and vomiting, oral mucositis and ovarian suppression with loss of fertility (Smith and deBoer 2000). Delivering adjuvant chemotherapy in the early stages of disease is difficult because benefits are delayed and most women are symptom free.

Hormone therapy

Most breast cancers retain oestrogen receptors and in these cancers oestrogen will retain control over the cancer cells (Chapman and Goodman 2000).

Tamoxifen

Tamoxifen, an anti-oestrogen drug, works by competing with oestrogen to bind to oestrogen receptors within breast cancer cells. Tamoxifen achieves the greatest benefit in patients with oestrogen receptor-positive tumours and is of little benefit in oestrogen-negative tumours. Clinical trials have shown tamoxifen to be most beneficial when taken as a 20-mg dose for 5 years. Unfortunately, tamoxifen also has a number of side effects which can seriously affect the quality of life of breast cancer patients: hot flushes, night sweats, altered libido, vaginal dryness and weight gain being some of the most distressing. Tamoxifen has also been shown to have a link to endometrial cancer in some women (Smith and deBoer 2000). Clinical trials are ongoing to compare tamoxifen with other anti-oestrogens in an attempt to reduce these side effects, although only 3% of patients stop treatment because of the side effects. A sensitive approach by the nurse and other health-care professionals can help women access supportive care and treatment in order to alleviate some of the symptoms and associated distress.

Oophorectomy

Oophorectomy is beneficial in women under 50 and can be achieved surgically, by radiation or hormonally. The side effects include induction of the menopause, vaginal dryness and hot flushes, and a link has been made to osteoporosis.

Although symptom management is cited by cancer patients as being key to cancer management, being treated with humanity and having someone to listen are seen as being just as important (DoH 2000). Whenever a nurse enters the breast cancer patient's journey, these skills are important and every patient will require different support at different times. An awareness of the possible side effects of surgery and adjuvant treatments and the ability to communicate effectively and sensitively cannot be underestimated.

Psychosocial issues

About 30% of women with breast cancer develop an anxiety state or depressive illness within a year of diagnosis, which is three or four times the norm in the rest of the population (Maguire 2000). Breast cancer patients often hide psychological problems because they do not think that they are acceptable; in this situation patients need permission to disclose how they are feeling. The psychological effects of having cancer can be a sense of loss, loss of health, opportunities, choice and control, uncertainty about the future, anxiety and depression (Grosser 2003).

After mastectomy 20–30% of problems may be related to body image and sexuality; however, immediate reconstruction may help reduce psychiatric morbidity as long as the patient is fully informed about the procedure and possible complications (Maguire 2000). Changes in sexuality after a breast cancer diagnosis depend on the woman's psychological health and how she viewed herself sexually before the diagnosis. Most health professionals still fail to address sexuality in the clinical setting and feel more comfortable focusing on treatment outcomes such as the management of side effects (Hordern 2000).

Social support is also associated with better adjustment and decreased emotional distress among patients with cancer. Social support, according to Lugton (1997), maintains identities for women wanting to get back to normal in their relationships and work as well as adapting to an uncertain future. Nurses play a key role in informal support systems, enabling women time to adjust and come to terms with their experience (Lugton 1997). Support groups are a good example of informal support and in some areas are very active.

Breast care specialist nurses have an important role to play as part of the multidisciplinary team caring for the patient. Research endorses the value of this specialist role particularly in identifying those women at risk of psychiatric morbidity (Maguire 2000).

The role of the nurse

A study by Wang et al. (1999) on the major concerns and needs of breast cancer patients highlighted the importance of information needs and empowerment for themselves and for their family; where this was provided in a sensitive environment, psychosocial problems were prevented.

Breast cancer is a frightening diagnosis for any woman and the importance of appropriate support at every stage cannot be overemphasized. According to the Royal College of Nursing (RCN 2002), the nurse's role is predominantly educational: encouraging women to be familiar with their breasts, offering both verbal and written information, being aware of the management of breast problems and informing women about the screening programme. The breast awareness 'five-point plan' advocates (Patnick 1995):

- knowing what is normal
- looking at and feeling the breasts
- knowing what changes to look for
- knowing what to do if a change is found
- attending for screening if over 50.

The role of the nurse is therefore to empower women by providing information, advice and support (Bailey 2000). Women need to be empowered to cope with the many life changes that face them and decisions that they need to make on their breast cancer journey (Fallowfield et al. 1994).

Conclusion

Research is ongoing in most areas of breast care, with choices to be made about surgical treatment and breast reconstruction, as well as treatments for local and systemic therapy. It is clear that supportive care is essential if women are to be empowered in order to make treatment decisions at a time when they are feeling less able to do so. Effective communication and supportive care are also of great importance to the long-term adjustment to treatment for breast cancer. A person's desire for autonomy may be less strong than the need for clear and accurate information (Fallowfield et al. 1994). Patients are clear about what they want from the nurse: a friend, confidant(e), explainer, comforter and counsellor, as well as a nurse (Bottomley and Jones 1997). Nurses must ensure that care is coordinated with the multidisciplinary team, using appropriate communication skills and resources, to deliver the highest standards of care.

References

Bailey K (2000) The nurse's role in promoting breast awareness. Nurs Stand 14(30): 34–6.
Bhakta P (1995) Asian women's attitudes to breast self examination. Nurs Times 91(8): 44–7.
Blamey RW, Wilson ARM, Patnick J (2000) Screening for breast cancer. In: Dixon JM (ed.), ABC of Breast Diseases, 2nd edn. London: BMJ Books, pp. 33–7.
Bottomley A, Jones L (1997) Breast cancer care: women's experience. Eur J Cancer Care 6: 124–32.
Bundred NJ, Morgan DAL, Dixon JM (2000) Management of regional nodes in breast cancer. In: Dixon JM (ed.), ABC of Breast Diseases, 2nd edn. London: BMJ Books, pp. 44–9.
Cancer Research UK (2004) www.cancerhelp.org.uk/help/default.asp?page3270
Carlisle D (2002) Cancer: the big picture. Nurs Times 98(35): 22–4.
Carroll S (1998) Breast cancer Part 2: management. Prof Nurse 13: 791–5.
Chapman D, Goodman M (2000) Breast cancer. In: Yarbro C, Frogge M, Goodman M, Groenwald S (eds) Cancer Nursing: Principles and practice, 5th edn. Boston, MA: Jones & Bartlett.
Cimprich B (1999) Pretreatment symptom distress in women newly diagnosed with breast cancer. Cancer Nurs 22: 185–94.
Dixon JM, Mansell RE (2000) Symptoms, assessment and guidelines for referral. In: Dixon JM (ed.), ABC of Breast Diseases, 2nd edn. London: BMJ Books, pp. 1–9.
Department of Health (2000) The NHS Cancer Plan: A plan for investment, a plan for reform. London: HMSO.
Fallowfield LJ, Hall A, Maguire P, Baum M, Hern RPA (1994) Psychological effects of being offered choice of surgery for breast cancer. BMJ 309: 448.
Grosser L (2003) The special needs of younger women. Cancer Nurs Pract 2(1): 13–14.
Hermon C, Beral V (1995) Breast cancer mortality rates are levelling off or beginning to decline in many Western countries: analysis of time trends; age cohort and age period models of breast cancer mortality in 20 countries. Br J Cancer 73: 955–60.
Hordern A (2000) Intimacy and sexuality for the woman with breast cancer. Cancer Nurs 23: 230–6.

Keeton S, McAloon L (2002) The supply and fitting of a temporary breast prosthesis. Nurs Stand 16(41): 43–6.

Lugton J (1997) The nature of social support as experienced by women treated for breast cancer. J Adv Nurs 25: 1184–91.

McPherson K, Steel CM, Dixon JM (2000) Breast cancer: epidemiology, risk factors and genetics. In: Dixon JM (ed.), ABC of Breast Diseases, 2nd edn. London: BMJ Books, pp. 26–32.

Maguire P (2000) Psychological aspects. In: Dixon JM (ed.), ABC of Breast Diseases, 2nd edn. London: BMJ Books, pp. 85–9.

Miller WR, Ellis I, Sainsbury JRC (2000) Prognostic factors. In: Dixon JM (ed.), ABC of Breast Diseases, 2nd edn. London: BMJ Books, pp. 78–84.

National Health Service Breast Screening Programme (1998) Quality Assurance Guidelines for Nurses in Breast Cancer Screening. Sheffield: NHSBSP

Nystrom R, Moss S, McGahan C, Quinn M, Babb P (2000) Effect of NHS breast screening programme on mortality from breast cancer in England and Wales, 1990–8: comparison of observed with predicted mortality. BMJ 321: 665–70.

Page DL, Steel CM, Dixon JM (2000) Carcinoma in situ and patients at high risk of breast cancer. In: Dixon JM (ed.), ABC of Breast Diseases, 2nd edn. London: BMJ Books, pp. 90–6.

Patnick J (1995) Giving the knowledge. Nurs Stand 9(26): 20–1.

Royal College of Nursing (2002) Breast Palpation and Breast Awareness: The role of the nurse. London: RCN.

Sainsbury JRC, Anderson TJ, Morgan DAL (2000) Breast cancer. In: Dixon JM (ed.), ABC of Breast Diseases, 2nd edn. London: BMJ Books, pp. 38–43.

Smith IE, deBoer RH (2000) Role of systemic treatment for primary operable breast cancer. In: Dixon JM (ed.), ABC of Breast Diseases, 2nd edn. London: BMJ Books, pp. 55–60.

Vogel W (2003) The advanced practice nursing role in a high risk breast cancer clinic. Oncol Nurse Forum 30(1) 115–22.

Wang X, Cosby L, Harris M, Liu T (1999) Major concerns and needs of breast cancer patients. Cancer Nurs 22: 157–63.

Chapter 5

Lung cancer

Lung cancer is the most common cancer in the world and is the second most common form of cancer in the UK, after breast cancer (Cancer Research UK 2004). There are 37 000 new cases of lung cancer in the UK each year (Cancer Research UK 2004). Although rising mortality from the disease has levelled off in men, it continues to rise in women and accounts for one in eight of all deaths from malignant disease; it has overtaken breast cancer as the number one killer in women (Myatt and Treasure 2002). Lung cancer occurs most frequently between the ages of 50 and 60 years; however, it is increasingly being seen in younger age groups (Garden et al. 2002). There is no effective screening test and a limited range of treatment options results in lung cancer having a generally poor prognosis (Lowden 1998). The 5-year overall survival rate for lung cancer patients is only 5.8% and only about 20% are alive a year after diagnosis (Thames Cancer Registry 1995). Sixty per cent of patients present in the late stages of the disease and up to 30% of patients undergoing surgery have undiagnosed metastases (Harpole 1995). Smoking has been identified as the main cause of lung cancer (Garden et al. 2002).

Anatomy and physiology

The lungs are two spongy cone-shaped organs situated in the thoracic cavity. They are separated by the heart and other structures. The lungs form part of the respiratory system whose organs include the nose, pharynx, larynx, trachea, bronchi and lungs.

The lungs act with the cardiovascular system to supply oxygen and remove carbon dioxide from the blood by the mechanism of breathing. They are protected by a double-layered serous membrane, the pleural membrane, the outer layer of which is attached to the wall of the thoracic cavity and the diaphragm, known as the parietal pleura. The inner layer or visceral pleura is attached to the lungs. The pleural cavity, which lies in between, contains a lubricating fluid secreted by the membranes (Tortora and Grabowski 2004). Deep grooves called fissures divide each lung into lobes: the right lung has three lobes and the left lung has two lobes (Figure 5.1). Each lung lobe is divided into smaller compartments called lobules which each contain a lymphatic vessel, an arteriole, a venule and a branch from a terminal bronchiole. The terminal bronchiole is part of the bronchiole tree which divides from the right and left bronchi, which in turn divide from the trachea. Each terminal bronchiole subdivides into microscopic branches called respiratory bronchioles, which divide further into alveolar ducts, alveolar sacs and alveoli (Tortora and Grabowski 2004). The exchange of gases occurs across a respiratory membrane, consisting of alveolar cells, basement membrane and endothelial cells of the capillary, during the mechanism of breathing.

Figure 5.1 Anatomy of the lungs

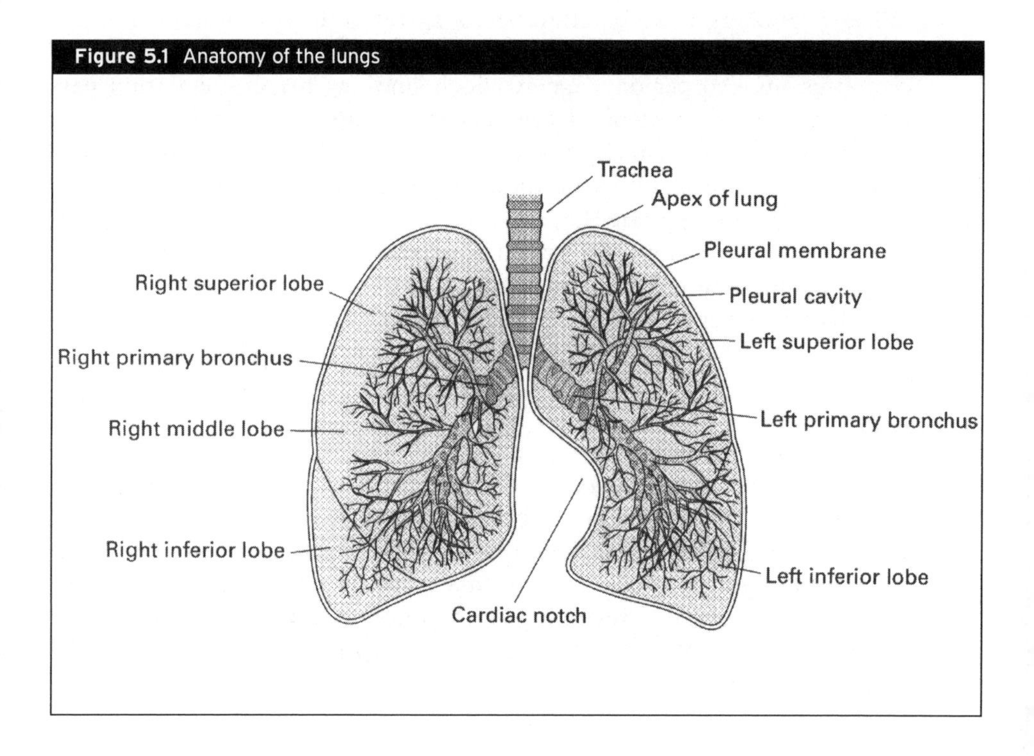

Breathing consists of inhalation and exhalation or the movement of air in and out of the lungs, moving from higher to lower pressure. Movement of the diaphragm and external intercostal muscles expands and decreases the volume of the lungs, which are under the control of the respiratory centre in the medulla oblongata area of the brain.

Risk factors

Smoking

Smoking is the major cause of lung cancer and is responsible for nine out of ten cases (Cancer Research UK 2004). Epidemiological studies have proved a causal link between lung cancer and smoking (Novello et al. 1991, Samet 1992, Zang and Wynder 1996) and it is well known that not only those who smoke are at risk (Cancer Research UK 2004). Hirayama (1981) demonstrated that non-smoking wives of husbands who smoked heavily had an increased risk of lung cancer. Similar results were found in studies of children and adults exposed to environmental tobacco smoke in their homes (Sandler et al. 1985). The risk of lung cancer development in heavy smokers is estimated to be 10–25 times the risk of non-smokers. The risk from smoking is determined by a number of factors: number of cigarettes smoked per day, age at which smoking began, inhalation patterns and the tar content of the cigarettes (Samet 1992). Studies have shown that reducing tar exposure can reduce the risk of lung cancer (Potanovitch 1993). Other studies, however, show that when smokers choose a low-tar cigarette they inhale more deeply thus negating the perceived benefits of smoking a low-tar cigarette (Wynder and Kabat 1988). Stopping smoking reduces risk. After 10 smoke-free years, the risk may be halved (Cancer Research UK 2004).

Diet

There is little evidence of a dietary cause for lung cancer; however, diets that are high in fruit and vegetables may be protective against lung cancer, whereas diets deficient in vitamin A appear to be associated with the disease. Despite this, chemoprevention trials with Vitamin A have shown no benefit in preventing lung cancer (Alpha-Tocopherol, Beta Carotene Cancer Prevention Study Group 1994, Cancer Research UK 2004).

Exposure to carcinogens

Exposure to asbestos, radon, chromium, nickel and inorganic arsenic compounds has been proved to increase an individual's risk of developing lung cancer (Ginsberg et al. 2001, Cancer Research UK 2004).

Social background

Lung cancer rates are strongly linked to socioeconomic deprivation, with those in the most deprived groups having rates two to three times higher than the least deprived groups. This reflects the smoking habits within these groups (Cancer Research UK 2004).

Family history

There is little evidence to show a genetic link for lung cancer.

Prevention

Smoking is the greatest avoidable risk factor for lung cancer, causing nine out of ten cases of the disease (DoH 2000, Cancer Research UK 2004). In the UK epidemiological research has shown that tobacco-related lung cancer deaths, over the next 50 years, will be influenced far more by the rate at which people are giving up smoking than by young people taking up the habit. Research is ongoing into the effectiveness of treatments to help smokers stop and into the general understanding about the addictive nature of tobacco (DoH 2000, Cancer Research UK 2004).

According to Cancer Research UK (2004) quitting is the best thing you can do for your health and not just in relation to lung cancer; smoking causes heart disease, stroke and emphysema, and can harm unborn babies and children who are exposed to passive smoke. For those who quit smoking:

- After 20 minutes: blood pressure and pulse return to normal
- After 8 hours: blood oxygen levels return to normal.
- After 24 hours: body is free of carbon monoxide
- After 3 years: risk of heart attack is same as that for non-smoker
- After 10 years: lung cancer risk is halved
- After 15 years: health is same as that of non-smoker.

Primary care trusts have taken the lead in smoking cessation programmes, including the appointment of health-care professionals to support those smokers wishing to quit. The government is also working with employers, local authorities, community groups, schools, churches, leisure facilities and minority ethnic groups to fund local alliances for action on smoking (DoH 1999).

Screening

In the early 1970s the National Cancer Institute's (NCI's) Early Lung Cancer Group screened 30 000 male smokers with chest radiographs and sputum cytology. Although lung cancers were detected more frequently at an early stage, long-term survival rates did not improve (Szabo et al. 1993). Low-dose spiral computed tomography (CT) can identify lung cancer in asymptomatic individuals at high risk. A large study is under way in the USA and a proposal for a trial in the UK is currently under consideration by the Medical Research Council (DoH 2000). At present there is no screening technique that is sensitive enough to be used for mass screening (DoH 2000).

The disease

Lung cancers can be broadly classified into two forms: small cell carcinomas and non-small cell carcinomas.

Non-small cell carcinomas

This classification is based on the characteristics of the tumour and its response to treatment (Kumar and Clark 1998). Non-small cell carcinomas are further divided into squamous cell carcinomas, adenocarcinomas and large cell carcinomas.

Squamous cell carcinomas arise from the cells lining the airways and account for about 30% of all lung cancers. This type of tumour is one of the two most commonly associated with smoking, the other being small cell carcinoma. Squamous cell carcinomas are usually found in the central part of the chest and tend to grow relatively slowly. They are the cancers that are most likely to remain centrally located.

Adenocarcinomas derive from mucus-producing cells and are the most common form of lung cancer found in non-smokers and women. About 30–40% of lung cancers are adenocarcinomas, and they have a higher tendency to metastasize than squamous cell carcinomas.

Large cell carcinomas are the least common form, accounting for about 10–15% of lung cancers. These cancers are also likely to metastasize.

Small cell carcinomas

Small cell carcinomas tend to originate in central locations and grow very rapidly. A large majority of patients with this type of cancer have metastatic disease. It is also known as oat cell carcinoma. It arises from endocrine cells in the lungs and secretes a number of polypeptide hormones, which lead to rapid cellular growth. It is considered a systemic disease and has previously been said to be the only one of the bronchial cancers that responds to chemotherapy, although research has been conducted that has sparked interest in treatment with platinum-based agents (Morgan 1996, Kumar and Clark 1998, Lowden 1998).

Signs and symptoms

The signs and symptoms of lung cancer arise from local intrathoracic and metastatic tumour growth, extrathoracic metastases and the indirect effects of the tumour. Tumour spread is via local invasion or the lymphatic system. Tumours can invade organs such as the pericardium, heart, oesophagus, chest wall or diaphragm (Quinn 1999). There are no signs or symptoms that are specifically diagnostic of lung cancer (Ginsberg et al. 2001). Some of the symptoms found in patients with lung cancer are also found in people who smoke or have other disorders, including upper respiratory infections. Signs and symptoms are related to the size and location of the primary tumour and to the presence of metastatic disease. Common symptoms include cough and haemoptysis. Wheezing and dyspnoea caused by airway occlusion may also occur. Some tumours may be asymptomatic and are picked up with a routine chest radiograph. If the malignancy is in a major airway, there may be a reflexive cough resulting from the stimulation of nerve endings. Airway occlusion can lead to a silent collapse of the lung (atelectasis) or infection, leading to pneumonia and a lung abscess. Pneumonia that fails to resolve is suspicious (Garden et al. 2002). The laryngeal nerve can be affected by the tumour and hoarseness can occur from paralysis of the vocal cords.

The phrenic nerve, which controls the movement of the diaphragm, may be affected, leading to a decrease in lung volume and ventilation. If the lymph nodes become enlarged in the mediastinum, they can compress the superior vena cava and cause engorgement of the face and arms (superior vena caval syndrome). This is a potential medical emergency. Dysphagia can occur if the oesophagus is involved. Bony metastases are common and can cause severe pain and pathological fractures (Kumar and Clark 1998). When the chest wall and ribs are invaded by the tumour, the brachial plexus may become involved – known as Pancoast's tumour, which can cause severe shoulder pain. Metastases most commonly affect the liver and hypercalcaemia can occur as a result of squamous cell carcinoma.

Fatigue, anorexia and weight loss can occur and cachexia, the result of malnutrition, increases the basal metabolic rate, leading to the breakdown of fat reserves and lean muscle mass which is a common side effect

(Lowden 1998). Metastases to the adrenal glands in small cell lung cancer can also occur (Cerosimo 2002).

Diagnosis

Complete medical history and physical examination may reveal signs and symptoms suggestive of lung cancer (Ginsberg et al. 2001):

- Any change in the amount or consistency of any sputum expectorated may be important
- Shortness of breath
- Wheezing
- Chest pain
- Blood in the sputum
- Frequent respiratory infections.

Patients should be asked whether they smoke or have been exposed to environmental toxins such as asbestos. Bone pain, weight loss and fatigue will increase the suspicion of lung cancer.

Chest radiograph

This may reveal a mass, enlarged lymph nodes, pleural effusion or collapsed lung. Chest CT or magnetic resonance imaging (MRI) may detect abnormalities suspicious of cancer.

Sputum samples

These are needed for cytological examination, with about 80% of tumours being diagnosed on sputum cytology (Cerosimo 2002). However, some small tumours and tumours that are not close to an airway may not shed cells into the airway, so they will not be diagnosed.

Bronchoscopy

A bronchoscopy can be performed, which is a useful diagnostic tool. Lesions in the bronchi can be sampled using forceps brushes and washings. Lung cancer is present in 90% of cases where a visible lesion is found. Only lesions located within the airways can be reached via a bronchoscope; others may be out of reach.

Another technique is a fine needle biopsy of a lesion in the lung or a lymph node or metastatic lesion. Needle biopsy is especially useful for lesions beyond the reach of a bronchoscope. Mediastinoscopy is used to look at the superior mediastinal nodes and is used to stage the disease.

Treatment

This can involve surgery, chemotherapy or radiotherapy. Before any treatment a patient should be assessed by a specialist radiotherapy team to enable the best treatment option to be chosen (Lowden 1998), and various staging investigations will be carried out to determine the type of tumour, and its extent and distribution (Kumar and Clark 1998).

Surgery

According to Morgan (1996), the complete resection of tumours remains the best chance of cure. However, even with apparently curative resections only 35–40% of patients survive 5 years after diagnosis (Garden et al. 2002). Only 20–25% of patients are eligible for surgical resection at the time of diagnosis (Nevidjon and Sowers 2000). Up to 30% of the less aggressive non-small cell lung cancers may be amenable to surgery and small cell lung cancers may be managed by surgery and chemotherapy, depending on the TNM (tumour, node, metastasis) classification. The surgical resection rates in the UK, at less than 10%, are lower than those in the USA and Europe, which are more than 20%.

The main aim of surgical treatment is the removal of the anatomical unit containing the tumour, which could be a segment, lobe or whole lung. The associated lymphatic drainage will also be removed. As many lung cancer patients are chronic smokers they are poor surgical candidates (Ruckdeschel 1995).

Radiotherapy

Radiotherapy may be used for patients who are not able to undergo surgery or in those where the tumour is surgically unresectable. It is generally used to help reduce symptoms of intrathoracic disease and metastases. It is an important part of the treatment of advanced small cell lung cancer because these cancers respond well to short courses of radiotherapy (MacBeth 1996). Most non-small lung cancers have poor radiosensitivity. Radiotherapy may be used before or after surgery to treat regional lymph nodes. However, data show that, although this may reduce local recurrence and prolong the disease-free survival period, overall survival is not prolonged (Payne 1994, Cerosimo 2002). Radiotherapy can also be used palliatively to help reduce tumour size, which helps to relieve symptoms such as haemoptysis, cough, dyspnoea, obstruction of the airways, chest pain and hoarseness. Bone metastases can be treated, helping to reduce bone pain. Radiotherapy is also used to relieve spinal cord compression and help prevent paralysis and superior vena caval obstruction. It can be used prophylactically in those patients at high risk of brain metastases.

Chemotherapy

Although unlikely to cure patients with advanced lung cancer, chemotherapy is useful for palliation of symptoms and as an aid to prolong survival. Small cell tumours metastasize early and are regarded as a systemic disease at the time of diagnosis. They are responsive to chemotherapy and single or combination therapies may be used. Although non-small cell lung cancer has been regarded as resistant to chemotherapy, research with platinum-based agents has increased interest in combined surgery and preoperative (neoadjuvant) or postoperative (induction) chemotherapy (Morgan 1996, Lowden 1998).

Psychosocial issues

Quality of life is defined as the impact of physical symptoms and side effects of treatment on a patient's functioning and well-being (Fergusson and Cull 1991). Nurses can play an important role by helping patients address the fears that surround being diagnosed with a potentially fatal disease. Given an opportunity, most patients will express their anger and frustration. Allowing them to talk without necessarily offering them answers can be beneficial (Quinn 1999).

As patients may experience distressing symptoms such as dyspnoea, fatigue and weight loss, they may be socially restricted and isolate themselves as a way of coping. If they smoke they may isolate themselves further for fear of criticism. This isolation will have a negative impact on their quality of life.

Social support is associated with better adjustment and decreased emotional distress and helps adaptation to a future of uncertainty. Nurses play an important role in support and can be effective in enabling adjustment (Lugton 1997).

The role of the nurse

Prevention of cancer is a major aim of *The NHS Cancer Plan* (DoH 2000). Smoking is the single greatest cause of preventable and early death in the UK (DoH 1999). *Smoking Kills* (DoH 1999) has three challenging targets to reduce smoking and in *The Health of the Nation* (DoH 1992) targets for lung cancer aim to reduce death rates from lung cancer by 2010. The report highlights the role of nurses, stating that they should be concerned with influencing individual behaviours via health promotion, education and screening (DoH 1992). Nurses should be trained to use effective interventions to reduce the uptake of smoking and aid smoking cessation (Melville and Eastwood 1998). Continued smoking after a cancer diagnosis is associated with decreased survival, increased risk of recurrence of a secondary tobacco-related cancer and postoperative morbidity, as well as increased side effects of chemotherapy and radiotherapy (Sarna 1999). Nurses can help coordinate care with members of the interdisciplinary team and keep the patient and the family informed. Providing end-of-life care will be an important role for the nurse because 90% of lung cancer patients die within 5 years of diagnosis. The nurse's role will encompass helping patients to adjust and adapt from controlling disease to symptom relief.

Conclusion

Lung cancer is the most common cancer in the world and also the most preventable (Cerosimo 2002, Cancer Research UK 2004). For those who contract lung cancer the prognosis is poor with only 10–15% of sufferers surviving more than 5 years after diagnosis (Garden et al. 2002). Smoking cessation and prevention are at the forefront of government strategies to reduce lung cancer-related morbidity and mortality. Health-care professionals have a vital part to play in educating and supporting people to quit smoking by offering clear information and working in partnership (DoH 2000, National Institute for Clinical Effectiveness or NICE 2004).

References

Alpha-Tocopherol, Beta Carotene Cancer Prevention Study Group (1994) The effect of Vitamin E and Beta-Carotene on the incidence of lung cancer and other cancers in male smokers. N Engl J Med 330: 1029–35.

Brogdon C (1998) Women and cancer. J Intraven Nurs 6: 344–55.

Cancer Research UK (2004) Lung Cancer: Briefsheet. London: Cancer Research UK.

Cerosimo RJ (2002) Lung cancer: A review. Am J Health Systems Pharmacol 59: 611–42.

Department of Health (1992) The Health of The Nation. London: HMSO.

Department of Health (1993) The Health of the Nation: Targeting Practice. The contribution of Nurses, Midwives and Health Visitors. London: HMSO.

Department of Health (1999) Smoking Kills. London: HMSO.

Department of Health (2000) The NHS Cancer Plan: A plan for investment, a plan for reform. London: Department of Health.

Doll R, Peto P (1996) Oxford Textbook of Medicine. Oxford: Oxford University Press.
Fergusson RJ, Cull A (1991) Quality of life measurements for patients undergoing treatment for lung cancer. Thorax 46: 671–5.
Garden OJ, Bradbury AW, Forsythe JLR (2002) Principles and Practice of Surgery, 4th edn. Edinburgh: Churchill Livingstone.
Ginsberg RJ, Vokes EE, Rosenzweig K (2001) Non-small cell lung cancer. In: De Vita VT, Hellman S, Rosenberg SA (eds), Cancer: Principles and practice of oncology, 6th edn. Philadelphia, PA: Lippincott, Williams & Wilkins, pp. 925–83.
Harpole DH (1995) Prognostic issues in non-small cell lung cancer. Chest 107(suppl 6): 267–9S.
Hirayama T (1981) Non-smoking wives of heavy smokers have a higher risk of lung cancer. BMJ 282: 183–5.
Kumar P, Clark M (1998) Clinical Medicine, 4th edn. Edinburgh: WB Saunders.
Laroche C, Wells F, Coulden R et al. (1998) Improving surgical resection rates in lung cancer. Thorax 53: 445–9.
Lowden B (1998) The care and treatment of lung cancer. Nurs Times 94(9): 61–2.
Lugton J (1997) The nature of social support as experienced by women treated for breast cancer. J Adv Nurs 25: 1184–91.
MacBeth F (1996) Radiotherapy in the treatment of lung cancer: indications and side effects. Br J Hosp Med 55: 639–642.
Melville A, Eastwood A (1998) A wider role in managing patients with lung cancer. Nurs Times 19(94): 33
Morgan WE (1996) The surgical management of lung cancer. Br J Hosp Med 55: 631–4.
Myatt R, Treasure T (2002) Lung cancer: the harsh reality. Cancer Nurs Pract 1(9): 10–11.
Myers MF (1994) How much investigation? In: Thatcher N, Spiros (eds), Perspectives in Lung Cancer. London: BMJ Publishing Group.
Nevidjon BM, Sowers KW (eds) (2000) A Nurse's Guide to Cancer Care. Philadelphia, PA: Lippincott.
National Institute for Clinical Effectiveness (2004) Improving Supportive and Palliative Care for Adults with Cancer. London: NICE.
Novello AC, Davis RM, Giovino GA (1991) The slowing of the lung cancer epidemic and the need for continued vigilance (Editorial). CA: Cancer J Clin 41: 133–5.
Payne PG (1994) Is preoperative or postoperative radiation therapy indicated in non-small cell cancer of the lung? Lung Cancer 10: 5202–12.
Potanovitch LM (1993) Lung cancer: prevention and detection update. Semin Oncol 9: 174–9.
Quinn S (1999) Lung cancer: the role of the nurse in treatment and prevention. Nurs Stand 13(41): 49–54.
Ruckdeschel JC (1995) Carcinoma of the lung. In: Ravel RE (ed.), Conn's Current Therapy. Philadelphia, PA: WB Saunders, pp. 156–162.
Samet JM (1992) The health benefits of smoking cessation. Med Clin North Am 76: 399–414.
Sandler DP, Wilcox AJ, Everson RB (1985) Cumulative effects of lifetime passive smoking on cancer risk. Lancet i: 312–15.
Sarna L (1999) Prevention: tobacco control and cancer nursing. Cancer Nurs 1: 21–28.
Szabo E, Birrer MJ, Mulshine JL (1993) Early detection of lung cancer. Semin Oncol 20: 374–82.
Thames Cancer Registry (1995) Prognostic issues in non-small cell lung cancer. Chest 6(suppl): 267S–69S.
Tortora GJ, Grabowski SR (2004) Introduction to the Human Body. New York: Wiley.
Wynder E, Kabat GC (1988) The effect of low yield cigarette smoking on lung cancer risk. Cancer 62: 1223–30.
Yarbro CH, Hansen Frogge M, Goodman M, Groenweld SL (eds) (2000) Cancer Nursing. Principles and practice, 5th edn. Sudbury, MA: Jones & Bartlett.
Zang EA, Wynder EL (1996) Differences in lung cancer risk between men and women. Examination of the evidence. J Natl Cancer Inst 88:183–92.

Chapter 6

Prostate cancer

Prostate cancer is the most common male cancer in many westernized countries and the second leading cause of cancer deaths in men. Over 27 000 new cases of prostate cancer were diagnosed in the UK in 2000, one in 20 cases occurring in the under-60 age group (Cancer Research UK 2004). The incidence of prostate cancer has increased steadily since 1970 and, according to the Cancer Research Campaign (CRC), this trend will continue upwards (DeVita et al. 2001, CRC 1997) and it is predicted that prostate cancer incidence will overtake that of lung cancer and become the most commonly diagnosed cancer in men by 2006 (*Everyman* 2002). Kirby (2000) describes the disease as an 'epidemic' in waiting and Holmberg (1998) believes that it is an important health problem with considerable social and economic consequences. Characteristically, it is a disease of older men, with 80% of diagnosed cases in men aged 65 years and over (Ofman 1993); it represents a growing health problem for society (Boyle 1996).

The increased incidence could be accounted for because there are newer methods of detecting the disease (Blandy and Fowler 1996) and as the longevity of the population increases morbidity and mortality from prostate cancer will continue to rise (Dearnaley 1994). Vetrosky (1997) believes that the increasing incidence is associated with increased public awareness of the disease. Peate (1998), however, believes that the increases are the result of a combination of factors, namely better and improved diagnostic tools, new reporting techniques, changing diet and lifestyle.

Prostate gland anatomy and physiology

The prostate gland is part of the male genital system. It is located inferior to the bladder and anterior to the rectum, and situated posterior to the symphisis pubis to which it is attached by connective tissue. The gland measures about 3 cm in diameter, weighs about 20 g and resembles a walnut in size and shape (Figure 6.1).

Figure 6.1 Position of the prostate gland

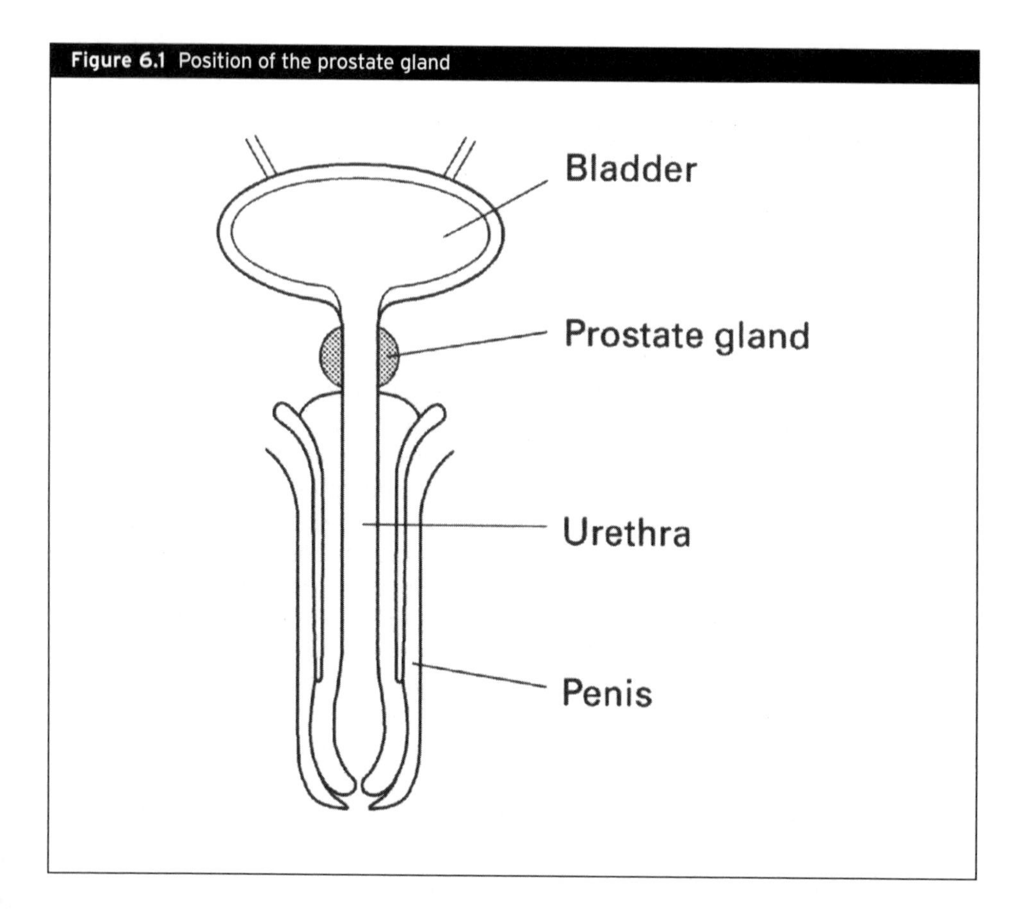

Laker and Leaver (1994) say that the size of the prostate varies. It increases in size around the age of puberty and then usually remains constant until the age of 45–50 years. At this time it may undergo varying degrees of enlargement stimulated by rising levels of the male hormone testosterone.

The prostate is composed of three distinct zones: peripheral, central and transitional zones. The physiological activity of the prostate depends on testosterone. Vetrosky (1997) says that the primary function of the prostate gland is in the protection against rising bacterial invasion of the bladder.

The prostate secretes a slightly acidic fluid, which is rich in enzymes such as acid phosphatase. This fluid makes up 13–33% of the volume of semen and contributes to the sperm motility and viability, although no definitive function has been proved (Blandy 1998).

Risk factors

Although the exact aetiology of prostate cancer is unknown, a number of risk factors that may predispose an individual to the development of prostate cancer are frequently proposed and these can be categorized into definitive, probable and potential risk factors.

Definitive risk factors

These are age, race and genetics:

- The incidence of prostate cancer increases sharply with age; by the age of 80 more than half of all men will have cancerous changes in the prostate (Cancer Research UK 2002).
- The highest risk has been reported in North America and northern European countries and the lowest in the Far East, with the risk proving greater in black than in white men. Men of African–American origin have rates of prostate cancer over 100 per 100 000 and in Asia it is 10 per 100 000. The risk factor rises in Asian men if they emigrate to the west (Department of Health or DoH 2000a).
- Research studies have suggested that there is an increase in a man's risk of developing prostate cancer when a first-degree relative (a father or brother) has been diagnosed with the disease (Carter 1992, 1993, McLellan and Norman 1995, Cancer Research UK 2004).

Probable risk factors

- These include diet and there appears to be a link between specific food types and prostate cancer, which tends to follow the general pattern for cancers. A correlation with dietary fat intake has been suggested, although the evidence in this area is inconclusive (Whitmore 1993, Giovanucci 1994, Cancer Research UK 2002). A decreased risk is associated with a high intake of vegetables rich in retinoids (the pigments found in yellow and red vegetables), particularly tomatoes. Fish may also be protective (Cohen et al. 2000, Terry et al. 2001, Cancer Research UK 2002).
- Prostate cancer is endocrine dependent and Ross and Bernstein (1992) demonstrate that black men have serum testosterone levels that are 15% higher than their white counterparts; this might account for the increased risk of black men developing prostate cancer. Ross and Bernstein (1992) showed that American men had different levels of testosterone-metabolizing enzymes than their Japanese counterparts, which could account for the differences in incidence among the two groups.

Potential risk factors

- These include vasectomy and certain environmental and occupational factors. Giovanucci (1994) suggests that men who have had a vasectomy have a greater predisposition to developing prostate cancer.
- A relationship between men working with cadmium in occupations such as welding and electroplating and the development of prostate cancer has been suggested (Lemen 1976, Hayes 1993).

Screening

Screening for prostate cancer is a controversial issue. Screening methods available can show false positives, which can lead to unnecessary investigation or even treatment for some men and be detrimental to their health (Austoker 1994, Jones 2003). Woolf (1997) says that routine screening is unwarranted when there is inconclusive evidence that this would detect early disease and that early detection would improve patient outcomes.

Screening techniques for prostate cancer include the following:

- Prostate-specific antigen (PSA) blood test: PSA is produced by the prostate gland and can be measured in the blood. PSA levels are usually raised in the presence of cancer; however, not all men with high PSA levels have prostate cancer and not all men with cancer have high PSA levels (Cancer Research UK 2004).
- Transrectal ultrasonography: this imaging technique involves an ultrasound probe inserted into the rectum to assess the size and shape of the prostate. This test is not patient friendly and has a high cost implication.
- Digital rectal examination (DRE): this test can detect lesions on the surface of the prostate, but it relies on a high degree of expertise by the examiner and can fail to detect small lesions (Kelly 2002).

There is currently no national screening programme in the UK; however, the Department of Health, in *The NHS Cancer Plan* (DoH 2000b), say that, once screening for prostate cancer has been agreed, it will be implemented. Currently men aged 50 years and over can request a test and should be given the necessary information about screening in order to decide for themselves which option to choose. Trials are currently under way with the National Cancer Institute and European Cancer programme to compare the screened and unscreened populations and subsequent survival. These studies involve 74 000 and 50 000 men. Results will be available in 2010 (Templeton 2003).

The disease

Pathophysiology

Prostate cancer is usually a slow growing malignancy (Held 1994, DoH 2000a), but if left untreated it grows progressively. Tumours most commonly arise in the peripheral zone of the prostate's glandular tissue. Prostate cancer is most often (99%) adenocarcinoma and about 1% a small cell cancer type (Murphy et al. 1994). The main methods of tumour spread are by intraprostatic growth, direct extension, lymphatic drainage and/or arterial venous blood flow. Most commonly it spreads to the skeleton and the lymph nodes but spread to the liver and lungs is common.

Symptoms

In the early stages it may be asymptomatic. As the cancer progresses symptoms may present. Many men present with similar symptoms to benign prostatic hypertrophy (BPH). This condition affects one-third of men over the age of 50 and is seen in most men over the age of 80. As stated earlier, the prostate enlarges as men age and when benign it is called benign hypertrophic disease (Billington 1999).

Symptoms of prostate cancer might include the following:

- Difficulty in passing urine: according to Peate (1998) the most frequent symptoms are frequency, urgency, dysuria, nocturia and a feeling of incomplete emptying of the bladder (National Institute for Clinical Excellence or NICE 2002).
- As many as 40% of men, however, present with metastatic disease (Kirby and Brawer 1996). Presenting symptoms of these men are usually bone pain or paraesthesia according to the individual situation. This is usually a result of the presence of bony metastases. In such cases the prostate cancer has usually remained asymptomatic until the tumour has metastasized. Some men, who may have had BPH-related symptoms for some time, may present with acute retention of urine and urgent admission is required (Jones 2003)

Diagnosis

When it is suspected that a man has prostate cancer, investigative tests need to be carried out. A full history is taken and a clinical examination performed. This will include a DRE, in which the doctor places a gloved finger into the patient's rectum to feel the prostate for any abnormalities.

Normally the prostate is smooth but, in prostate cancer, a hard nodule may be felt or the prostate may be enlarged and hard and craggy to the touch. A lack of mobility is often observed as a result of adhesion to surrounding tissues. However, according to Smith and Catalonia (1995), the DRE is subject to considerable interexaminer variability, which might result in false-positive diagnoses of prostate cancer. Such diagnoses might be made in the presence of conditions such as BPH, prostatitis or ejaculatory duct abnormalities (Kelly 2002).

Blood tests are conducted to confirm a suspected diagnosis of prostate cancer. The levels of PSA are measured. PSA is an enzyme produced by the epithelial cells of the prostate with the function of liquefying the ejaculate. The recommended reference range for PSA in a healthy individual is 0–4.0 ng/ml. Although a raised PSA can be indicative of prostate cancer, it can also be present in many benign prostatic conditions (Waxman and Sheer 1995). PSA alone is an inadequate tool for early detection of prostate cancer because a significant number of men with later evidence of malignancies have a PSA that is classed as being within normal limits, and as many as 20% of men carry mutations in the genes that control PSA levels, giving rise to high PSA readings without the presence of a tumour.

If abnormalities are found through DRE and the PSA is raised, the patient may be considered for a transrectal biopsy of the prostate with ultrasound guidance. Measurement of the tumour is possible and Kirby and Brawer (1996) state that this is the gold standard imaging technique for staging prostate cancer.

Grading and staging of prostate cancer

When prostate cancer is diagnosed assessment of the extent or staging of the tumour is the best predictor of prognosis. Prostate cancer is staged using the TNM (tumour, nodes, metastases) system that was developed by the American Joint Committee for Cancer (1997). The stages reflect the clinical progression of the disease. Grading of the tumour is also essential because treatment is often based on this information. The Gleason (1974) system is the most widely accepted, which is based on how differentiated a tumour is, with prognosis worsening with the loss of glandular differentiation.

Bone scan

This will identify the presence of bone metastases. Prostate cancer spreads primarily to the bony pelvis, femur and lower spine (Blandy and Fowler 1996).

Magnetic resonance imaging/computed tomography

Magnetic resonance imaging (MRI) and computed tomography (CT) are used to identify the spread of the cancer outside the prostate capsule.

Treatments

Currently, there is no agreement about the most effective treatment for prostate cancer that is confined to the prostate gland (NICE 2002). Management of the disease includes the following.

Active monitoring

In active monitoring, the patient does not receive any immediate treatment. This is usually employed in a man who is aged over 70 years with a low-grade lesion. The treatment is based on the thought that many men will die from causes other than their prostate cancer. PSA levels will be checked regularly and treatment started when symptoms occur or where PSA levels indicate that the disease may be advancing. Dearnaley (1994) suggests that there is no compelling evidence that watching and waiting until the disease is progressing produces inferior patient outcomes than active intervention. Watchful waiting is considered a reasonable choice of treatment for all men with a well-to-moderately differentiated cancer and a life expectancy of fewer than 10 years. Despite this many men are reluctant to accept conservative management (Donovan et al. 1999).

Surgical intervention

If the tumour is clinically localized and the man is expected to have a life expectancy of more than 10 years, a radical prostatectomy is considered. Long-term prognosis after radical prostatectomy is good, with 85% of patients remaining tumour free at 10 years (Walsh and Ford 1994). With this procedure, there is a risk of urinary incontinence, erectile dysfunction and impotence (NICE 2002).

Radiotherapy

Radiotherapy can be offered for both curative and palliative purposes. It is advantageous to those who are unsuitable for surgery. The side effects of radiotherapy include urinary frequency, incontinence, rectal irritation, diarrhoea and tiredness. Palliatively it can be used in the presence of bony metastases, pathological fractures or spinal cord compression. Internal radiotherapy via the means of brachytherapy is another treatment option. Theoretically, brachytherapy can deliver a greater amount of radiation to the prostate gland and a lesser dose to the surrounding organs than external beam radiation; however, it is available at only a few hospital trusts within the UK. This treatment is potentially curable, involves one stage of treatment and has a short hospitalization; known side effects include bowel problems, bleeding secondary to radiation proctitis, prostatitis, acute retention of urine and a 21% risk of impotence (D'Amico 2002).

Hormone manipulation therapy

More than half of men with prostate cancer have locally advanced or metastatic disease at diagnosis and cannot be cured by either radiotherapy or surgery (Soloway 1998). Treatment at this stage must be considered palliative. The mainstay of treatment for these men is often hormone manipulation therapy (HMT), the aim of which is to inhibit the production of testosterone because this hormone aids the growth of prostate cancer. This can be achieved via surgical or medical methods.

Surgical method

Bilateral orchidectomy (removal of both testes) decreases the testosterone level by 90–95% and is effective immediately (Miakowski 1999).

Medical method

This has become a more acceptable treatment option for patients with locally advanced prostate cancer and offers comparable efficacy to the surgical method. This treatment downstages the tumour through a reduction in the amount of testosterone in the body, which causes either growth of the tumour to slow down or the size of the tumour to shrink. HMT reduces the tumour and slows the cancer progression in around 80% of men with locally advanced disease (Kirby 2000). The treatment is administered via a single quarterly depot injection. Initially this can cause a transient increase in testosterone and lead to increased bone pain or problems with urinary function. This effect is known as a tumour flare. Other side effects include impotence, hot flushes, decreased libido, diarrhoea, and nausea and vomiting.

Anti-androgens can also be used; these drugs block the effect of testosterone on the body. Side effects may include breast tenderness and swelling, stomach upsets and diarrhoea. The libido may be maintained. If prostate cancer does not respond to these treatments then oestrogen can be used. This female hormone is used as a last resort because of the risk of the man developing cardiovascular problems.

Psychosocial issues

After a diagnosis of prostate cancer, patients experience physical and psychosocial problems and require practical advice and emotional support to help them cope with this condition. Any diagnosis of cancer can produce reactions and feelings of anxiety and depression. Fear of death, of the unknown and of altered body image can also occur (Heidrich and Ward 1992). As prostate cancer affects body functions that are usually kept private, it can lead to feelings of embarrassment and have an adverse effect on sexuality (Moore and Estey 1999). Urinary incontinence, which can occur after treatment for prostate cancer, can cause embarrassment and affect emotional and social well-being.

Sexual dysfunction
Impotence may result after prostatic surgery or radiotherapy. It occurs when nerve supply to the pelvis is damaged or the blood supply to the penis is affected. Sexual drive or desire can be affected by hormone therapy and bilateral orchidectomy (Fan 2002).

The role of the nurse

Individuals undergoing all types of treatment for prostate cancer can experience problems that have a significant influence on their quality of life. The nurse has an important role to play in helping. Tools are available that enable the nurse to assess such factors as symptoms, quality of life and psychological well-being. An example of this is the European Organisation for Research and Treatment of Cancer's Quality of Life Questionnaire (EORTC QLQ – Aaronsen 19990). This questionnaire measures the psychological and physical distress associated with cancer. Borghede and Sullivan (1996) developed a 20-item prostate cancer supplement to allow this instrument to be used with prostate cancer patients. The information needs of clients must also be assessed because information is often viewed as an essential form of support (Fan 2002). The importance of addressing such needs has been emphasized in *The NHS Cancer Plan* (DoH 2000b). Moore and Estey (1999) found that men had a lack of knowledge about their post-surgery recovery period, specifically relating to catheter care, postoperative pain, incontinence and erectile dysfunction. Effective liaison between ward staff and the specialist nurse can help address these issues.

Conclusion

Prostate cancer is a life-threatening disease that is not curable but is controllable with treatment. It is the most common male cancer in many westernized countries and the second most common cancer from which men die (Everyman 2002). The incidence has risen steadily over the years. Although the exact aetiology is unknown, some factors increase the risk, namely age and race. Routine screening for the disease is not undertaken and a variety of treatments is available. The treatments can cause distressing side effects; however, addressing the psychological needs of patients can bring about an improvement in symptoms and aid psychological adjustment, helping to improve quality of life for patients (Fan 2002). The nurse has a key role to play by thoroughly assessing patient needs, involving patients and carers in all aspects of care and liaising with the multidisciplinary team.

References

Aaronsen NK (1990) Quality of life research in cancer clinical trials: a need for common rules and language. Oncology 4: 59–66.
American Joint Committee for Cancer (1997) Cancer Staging Manual, 5th edn. Philadelphia, PA: Lippincott Raven.
Austoker J (1994) Screening for ovarian, prostatic and testicular cancers. BMJ 309: 315–20.
Billington A (1999) Prostate disease. Nurs Stand 13(25): 49–53.
Blandy J (1998) Lecture Notes on Urology, 5th edn. Oxford: Blackwell Science.
Blandy J, Fowler C (1996) Urology, 2nd edn. London: Blackwell Science.
Borghede G, Sullivan M (1996) Measurement of quality of life in localised prostatic cancer patients treated with radiotherapy: development of a prostate cancer specific module supplementing the EORTC QLQ 30. Qual Life Res 5: 212–21.
Boyle P (1996) Prostate cancer: the threat to health and strategies for control. In: Peeling W (ed.), Questions and Uncertainties in Prostate Cancer. Oxford: Marston Book Services.
Cancer Research Campaign (1997) The Challenge We Face: The latest cancer statistics. London: CRC.
Cancer Research UK (2002) Prostate Cancer: Briefsheet. London: Cancer Research UK.
Cancer Research UK (2004) Prostate Cancer: Briefsheet. London: Cancer Research UK.
Carter B (1992) Hereditary prostate cancer: epidemiologic and clinical features. J Urol 150: 797–802.
Carter B (1993) Mendelian inheritance of familial prostate cancer. Proc Natl Acad Sci USA 89: 3367–71.
Cohen JH, Kristal AR, Stanford JL (2000) Fruit and vegetable intakes and prostate cancer risk. J Natl Cancer Instit 92(1): 61–8.
D'Amico A (2002) Radiation therapy for prostate cancer. In: Walsh PC (ed.), Campbell's Urology, 8th edn. Philadelphia, PA: Saunders, pp. 3147–70.
Dearnaley D (1994) Cancer of the prostate. BMJ 308: 780–4.
Department of Health (2000a) NHS Prostate Cancer Programme. London: HMSO.

Department of Health (2000b) The NHS Cancer Plan: A plan for investment, a plan for reform. London: HMSO.

DeVita V, Hellman S, Rosenberg SA (2001) Cancer: Principles and practice of oncology, 6th edn. Pittsburgh, PA: Lippincott.

Donovan JL, Frankel SJ, Faulkner A, Selley S, Gillatt D, Hamdy FC (1999) Dilemmas in treating early prostate cancer: the evidence and a questionnaire survey of consultant urologists in the United Kingdom. BMJ 318: 299–300.

Everyman (2002) Prostate Cancer: www.icr.ac.uk/everyman/about/prostate html (last accessed 16 May 2004).

Fan A (2002) Psychological and psychosocial effects of prostate cancer. Nurs Stand 17(13): 33–7.

Giovanucci E (1994) A prospective study of dietary fat and risk of prostate cancer. JAMA 271: 498–500.

Gleason D (1974) Prediction of prognosis for prostatic adenocarcinoma by combined histologic grading and clinical staging. J Urol 111: 58–64.

Hayes R (1993) Vasectomy and prostate cancer in US blacks and whites. Am J Epidemiol 137: 263–9.

Heidrich S, Ward S (1992) The role of the self in adjustment to cancer in elderly women. Oncol Nurs Forum 19: 1491–6.

Held J (1994) Cancer of the prostate: treatment and nursing implications. Oncol Nurs Forum 21: 1517–29.

Holmberg H (1998) Economic evaluation of screening for prostate cancer: a randomised population based programme during a 10 year period in Sweden. Health Policy 45: 133–47.

Jones A (2003) Prostate cancer – an overview. Cancer Nurs Pract 2: 131–8.

Kelly D (1998) Survival tactics. Nurs Times 94(22): 27–8.

Kelly D (2002) The implications of improvements in screening for prostate cancer. Prof Nurse 17: 605–8.

Kirby R (2000) The Prostate. Small gland, big problem. Oxford: Prostate Research Campaign UK.

Kirby R, Brawer MK (1996) Fast Facts: Prostate cancer, 4th edn. Oxford: Health Press.

Laker C, Leaver R (1994) Urological cancer. In: Laker C (ed.), Urological Nursing. Harrow: Scutari Press.

Lemen R (1976) Cancer mortality among cadmium production workers. Ann NY Acad Sci 271: 273–9.

McLellan D, Norman R (1995) Hereditary aspects of prostate cancer. Can Med Assoc J 153: 895–900.

Miakowski C (1999) Prostate cancer. In: Miakowski C, Buschell P (eds), Oncology Nursing: Assessment and clinical care. London: Mosby.

Moore K, Estey A (1999) The early postoperative concerns of men after radical prostatectomy. J Adv Nurs 29: 1121–9.

Murphy GP, Busch C, Abrahamsson PA, McNeal JE, Miller GJ, Mostofi FK, Nagle RB, Nordling S, Parkinson C et al. (1994) Histopathology of localized prostate cancer. Consensus conference on Diagnosis and Prognostic Parameters in Localised Prostate Cancer. Scandinavian Journal Urology & Nephrology Supplementum. 162: 7–42; disscussion 115–27.

National Institute for Clinical Excellence (2002) Improving Outcomes in Urological Cancers. London: NICE.

Ofman U (1993) Psychosocial and sexual implications of genitourinary cancers. Semin Oncol Nurs 9: 286–92.

Peate I (1998) Cancer of the prostate 1: promoting men's health care needs. Br J Nurs 7(3): 152–8.

Ross RK, Bernstein L (1992) 5-Alpha-reductase activity and risk of prostate cancer among Japanese and US white and black males. Lancet 339: 887–9.
Smith D, Catalonia W (1995) Inter examiner variability of digital rectal examination in detecting prostate cancer. Urology 45: 70–74.
Soloway M (1998) Combined androgen blockade an optimal therapy for minimally advanced prostate cancer? Br J Urol 81: 87–95.
Templeton H (2003) The management of prostate cancer. Nurs Stand 17(21): 45–53.
Terry P, Lichenstein P, Feychting M, Ahlbom A (2001) Fatty fish consumption and risk of prostate cancer. Lancet 357: 1764–6.
Vetrosky D (1997) Prostate cancer: pathology, diagnosis and management. Clinicians Rev 7(5): 79–100.
Walsh M, Ford P (1994) New Rituals for Old: Nursing through the looking glass. Oxford: Butterworth Heinemann.
Waxman J, Sheer D (1995) Is prostate cancer worth diagnosing? BMJ 346: 1177–8.
Whitmore W (1993) Management of clinically localised prostate cancer. JAMA 269: 2676–7.
Woolf S (1997) Should we screen for prostate cancer? BMJ 314: 789–990.

Chapter 7

Gynaecological cancers

Gynaecological cancers are not the most common cancers in women although they do carry a heavy physical and psychological burden (Tabano et al. 2002). Quality of life can be severely affected by the loss of fertility, physical disfigurement and sexual change that can be brought about by the cancer and its treatment. In this chapter we discuss the common gynaecological cancers, namely cervical, uterine, endometrial and ovarian.

Cervical cancer

Each year there are over 3200 new cases of cervical cancer in the UK – 2% of cases of new cancer diagnoses. It is the second most common cancer in women under the age of 35 (Cancer Research UK 2004). Cervical cancer does not develop suddenly and there is usually a period when some of the cells lining the cervix develop abnormal changes, which can give rise to cervical cancer later on. These changes can be picked up through screening. The UK has seen a 26% decrease in the incidence of invasive cervical cancer over the past 5 years (Fischer 2002).

Anatomy and physiology of the cervix

The cervix forms the lower part of the uterus and lies partly in the upper vagina and partly in the retroperitoneal space, behind the bladder and in front of the rectum. The squamous epithelium of the vagina and ectocervix meets the columnar epithelium of the uterine cavity and the endocervix at the squamocolumnar junction or transformation zone. The transformation zone is considered to be the usual site of cervical cancer (Royal College of Nursing or RCN 1999).

Risk factors

The primary risk factor appears to be exposure to the human papilloma virus (HPV). There are many strains of HPV; some types can cause warts whereas others are known as high-risk types because they can cause abnormalities in the cervical cells and cervical cancer (Cancer Research UK 2004). The virus is present in almost all cervical cancers (NHS Cervical Screening Programme or NHSCSP 2000, Butcher 2001). The classic risk factors that have previously been identified are: young age at first intercourse, increased number of sexual partners, high parity, race and low socioeconomic status. All appear to be linked to sexual behaviour and exposure to the HPV (Janicek and Averette 2001). Cigarette smoking has also been identified as a risk factor with cigarette carcinogens being identified in the cervical mucosa (Janicek and Averette 2001).

Screening

Cervical screening identifies cervical abnormalities that, if left untreated, may develop into cervical cancer. It is not a test for cancer. Screening was first introduced in the late 1960s and in 1988 a comprehensive call-and-recall system was introduced. All women aged 20–49 are invited for a smear test at least once every 3 years and those aged 50–64 are invited at least once every 5 years. The coverage rate of the screening programme in the UK has gone up to a national average of 85% with 4 million women benefiting from screening. The death rate from cervical cancer has been falling by 7% a year (Department of Health or DoH 2000). According to the Department of Health the screening process is a difficult, repetitive task. Laboratories are stretched and in some places there are long delays in getting smear test results. New developments in technology may help address these problems and, over the last 2 years, the Pathology Modernisation Fund has allocated over £250 000 to cervical cytology laboratories.

The NHS Cancer Plan (DoH 2000) set out action to support and develop NHS staff. A four-tier skill-mix model is under development, which will encompass all grades of staff and will explore the potential for an advanced practitioner grade (DoH 2000). Certain groups of people have particular needs in relation to cervical screening. Women from minority ethnic groups often do not come forward for cervical screening. Culturally sensitive information and different approaches to giving information can often improve the accessibility of screening to these groups. Women with learning disabilities have been identified as not having the information or support that they need to decide whether or not to attend for cervical screening. The Department of Health established a working group, including women with learning disabilities, to draw up good practice guidance and materials for women and their families, supporters and health professionals (DoH 2000).

Pathophysiology

Since the introduction of colposcopy in 1925 and the pap smear in 1941, it is well established that cervical cancer is preceded by a preinvasive condition known as squamous intraepithelial lesion or cervical intraepithelial neoplasia. Over a period of time this preinvasive condition progresses to carcinoma *in situ* and then invasive cervical cancer (Fischer 2002). Histologically 80–90% of cervical tumours are squamous and 10–20% adenocarcinoma. The remainder are made up of other types, including adenosquamous, glassy cell, sarcoma and melanoma (RCN 1999).

Symptoms

Initially the patient may just have a watery, blood-stained, vaginal discharge (Moore-Higgs 2000). If this is not treated, the bleeding will become more frequent and heavier, especially after sexual intercourse and manipulation of the cervix. The patient may present with anaemia as the tumour becomes bigger; areas of it become necrotic and a foul-smelling discharge becomes apparent. As the tumour spreads, it will produce additional symptoms, which may be flank and sciatic pain; the tumour can extend into the bladder and bowel, and the patient may have pain or bleeding from that area. The patient may present with a deep vein thrombosis because there is compression of the vascular or lymphatic channels in the groin from enlarged lymph nodes (Fischer 2002). Visually the cancer may not be visible; however, the cervix may be enlarged. The cervix may appear to have a large barrel shape or an ulcerating lesion may appear (Fischer 2002).

Diagnosis

As previously discussed, the classic screening tool is a pap smear. Once an abnormality is suspected a colposcopy is performed, which is the examination of the cervix under magnification. It is an essential part of the NHSCSP and plays a central role in the management of premalignant disease (Jolley 2004).

Staging

The staging of cervical cancer is performed clinically rather than surgically. Staging is based on physical examination. A chest radiograph is performed to rule out the spread of cancer to the lung. Colposcopy with a biopsy of suspicious lesions, cystoscopy and proctosigmoidoscopy are performed to identify whether the disease has spread to the bladder or bowel; an intravenous urogram or other radiological imaging of the renal tract may also be carried out (Lamb and Moore 1997). Magnetic resonance imaging (MRI) may also be performed.

Patients are staged according to the International Federation of Gynaecology and Obstetrics guidelines (Fischer 2002):

- Stage I: disease is confined to the cervix.
- Stage II: disease where the cancer extends beyond the cervix but has not extended to the pelvic side wall.
- Stage III: disease has extended to the pelvic side wall.
- Stage IV: disease has spread to another organ such as the bowel or bladder.

Treatments

The definitive treatment for invasive cancer of the cervix involves surgery or radiotherapy, or a combination of both. Treatment will depend on the stage, size and histology of the patient. Patient fitness will also need to be taken into account. In general, comparable survival rates are seen with both treatment options (Blake et al. 1998). Surgery has advantages over radiotherapy in early disease, especially in the younger patient: treatment time is shorter, ovarian function is preserved and sexual morbidity reduced. Patients appear to be more accepting of this treatment

Radical hysterectomy or Wertheim's hysterectomy may be performed depending on the staging of the disease. The ovaries can be preserved in premenopausal women.

Radiotherapy is a treatment of choice for women with more advanced disease, those with poor prognosis or those who are not fit enough for surgery.

Chemotherapy is generally used to palliate symptoms or reduce the size of tumour and metastatic deposits before surgery or radiotherapy (RCN 1999).

Sexual issues

Research indicates that about 50% of women treated for gynaecological cancer have some sexual dysfunction as they recover and become cancer survivors (Anderson and Lutgendorf 1997).

Problems of sexual dysfunction include loss of sexual desire, decreased arousal, dyspareunia and difficulty achieving orgasm (Rako 1996). A high percentage of these problems is caused by a drop in hormonal levels as a result of surgery, radiotherapy or chemotherapy. If a woman has aggressive or radical surgery this will also impact on sexual function. Symptoms of the cancer or treatment, such as chronic fatigue, nausea, diarrhoea, altered genital appearance, vaginal dryness, pain, hair loss, tender scars or a stoma, can make sexual activity difficult, leaving individuals feeling asexual (Tabano et al. 2002).

Ovarian cancer

Ovarian cancer has been called the 'disease that whispers' or the 'silent killer' because symptoms were thought not to be apparent until the cancer had spread outside the ovary. However, according to Martin (2002) a large survey of women with ovarian cancer confirmed that most women are symptomatic but frequently have delays in diagnosis (Goff et al. 2000).

Ovarian cancer is the fourth most common cancer among women in the UK and the second most common gynaecological cancer (Bicheno 2004). Each year there are about 6800 new cases (Cancer Research UK 2004). It is the fifth leading cause of cancer death worldwide and carries one of the highest death:case ratios for any malignancy (Bowes and Butler 2002, Martin 2002).

Anatomy and physiology

The ovaries are two almond-shaped organs located on either side of the uterus. They produce eggs and the female hormones that both regulate the menstrual cycle and are responsible for female body characteristics. The ovaries change shape and position with the monthly cycle over a woman's lifetime (Martin 2002). About 90% of ovarian cancers form in the cells that line the ovaries (Cancer Research UK 2004).

The risk of ovarian cancer increases with age. Most ovarian cancers occur in women after they have gone through the menopause and half of them occur in women over the age of 65 years (Cancer Research UK 2004). Survival rates vary; women with stage I ovarian cancer have a 60–90% chance of surviving the disease for 5 years whereas women with stage III disease have only a 5–50% chance of 5-year survival (Martin 2002).

Risk factors

The factors that lead to ovarian cancer are not known, but factors associated with the risk include the following.

Family history

Most cases occur in women who do not have a family history although about 10% of cases occur in women with family histories (Claus et al. 1996). The risk of developing ovarian cancer is increased if there is a first-degree relative, i.e. mother, sister, daughter, who has or has had the disease, especially if they developed it at a young age. In general, the closer the degree of relative and the younger the relative age at diagnosis the greater the risk (Martin 2002, Cancer Research UK 2004). Three hereditary cancer syndromes are known in which ovarian cancer syndrome is a component: breast–ovarian cancer syndrome, site-specific ovarian cancer syndrome and hereditary non-polyposis colorectal cancer (Martin 2000).

Childbearing and menstrual history

Women who have never been pregnant are more likely to develop ovarian cancer than women who have had children. Women who start their periods at a young age, have the first child after the age of 30 and/or go through the menopause after the age of 50 may have an increased risk. Breast-feeding slightly lowers the risk (Cancer Research UK 2004).

Oral contraceptives

Women who have taken oral contraceptives have a lower risk of ovarian cancer (Cancer Research UK 2004).

Personal history of breast cancer

Women who have had breast cancer have a slightly greater risk of developing ovarian cancer, because they may carry mutations of the *BRCA-1* or *BRCA-2* gene.

Some evidence indicates that chronic inflammatory processes may be related to ovarian cancers. Things that may cause inflammation are use of talcum powder around the perineal area, asbestos exposure, endometriosis and pelvic inflammatory disease (Martin 2002).

New research indicates that use of aspirin or non-steroidal anti-inflammatory agents may reduce the risk of cancer and, although not definitive, one ovarian study seemed to suggest that regular aspirin could be inversely associated with the risk of ovarian cancer (Akhmedkhanov et al. 2001). Protective measures include tubal ligation and hysterectomy (Martin 2002).

Screening and prevention

According to Martin (2002) the area of prevention and early detection is the one that has deficiencies. The incidence of ovarian cancer is very low and there are no data to support general population screening. There is at present no screening test that is reliable enough to use for ovarian cancer in the general population. However, it may be recommended for high-risk individuals.

Clinical trials are currently investigating screening. The trials are looking at screening in women at high risk of cancer of the ovary and women in general. There are two main tests being used in the screening trials: a blood test for CA-125 and transvaginal ultrasonography.

Blood test

The CA-125 blood test has been in use for over 20 years. CA-125 is known as a tumour marker for ovarian cancer. A tumour marker is a chemical that is given off by cancer cells and circulates in the bloodstream. Women with ovarian cancer tend to have higher levels of CA-125 in their blood than women who do not have ovarian cancer. However, there are difficulties with this test in that only about 85% of all women who have cancer of the ovary have a raised CA-125. Only 50% of women with early stage ovarian cancer have raised CA-125 and women with other conditions can also have raised levels of CA-125 (Cherry and Vacchiano 2002). Clearly, if levels can be raised in non-cancer conditions this could lead to a great deal of anxiety among women.

Transvaginal ultrasonography

This is done by putting the ultrasound probe into the vagina. It is generally agreed that transvaginal ultrasonography provides better visualization of the ovaries (Cherry and Vacchiano 2002). However, it can be difficult to tell whether a cancer or a cyst is present (Cancer Research UK 2004).

Currently trials are under way looking at screening for ovarian cancer. The first trial called UKTOCS (UK Trial for Ovarian Cancer Screening) is looking at screening in the general population and 200 000 women have been included. The trial consists of three groups:

- Group 1 have yearly CA-125 blood tests and, if abnormal, a transvaginal ultrasonography.
- Group 2 have yearly ultrasonography and, if abnormal, a blood test for CA-125.
- Group 3 have no screening.

A second trial, the UKFOCSS (UK Familial Ovarian Cancer Screening Study), is looking at screening for those with a family history of the disease (Cancer Research UK 2004).

Women at higher than average risk of getting the disease, i.e. having two or more relatives on the same side of the family with breast or ovarian cancer, diagnosed at a young age, could still be offered screening. Women are advised to visit their GP and be referred to the genetics screening centre; if appropriate, women will be listed on the UK Familial Ovary Cancer Register and, when the trial opens, they may be asked to join this second trial (Cancer Research UK 2004).

Prophylactic surgery

This is the removal of healthy, at-risk organs to reduce the risk of developing cancer. For women at risk of ovarian cancer, the options available vary from tubal ligation (tying of the fallopian tubes) to bilateral salpingo-oophorectomy (removal of both fallopian tubes and ovaries) and could include a total hysterectomy (removal of uterus). After removal of the ovaries, studies show a 67% reduction in risk for ovarian cancers. It is important to note that removal of the ovaries does not offer complete protection (Cherry and Vacchiano 2002).

Pathophysiology

The cell of origin classifies ovarian cancer. There are three major pathological categories of ovarian tumours with over 30 subtypes. The three main categories are epithelial, accounting for 85–90% of tumours, sex-cord stromal and germ-cell tumours (Anderson et al. 1997).

Symptoms

Women with ovarian cancer experience symptoms, most of which relate to abdominal bloating or gastrointestinal disturbances. Although women with early stage disease are less likely to have symptoms, only 11% reported that they had none at all (Goff et al. 2000). Symptoms include:

- increased abdominal size
- abdominal bloating
- fatigue
- abdominal pain
- indigestion
- urinary frequency
- pelvic pain
- urinary frequency
- constipation.

Diagnosis

A full medical history of the patient and the family will be taken and a pelvic examination performed. The patient will be referred to a specialist and further tests will be performed. These may include ultrasonography, CT or MRI, chest radiograph, intravenous urogram and laparoscopy (Cancer Research UK 2004).

Treatments

Surgery is the initial treatment for most women with ovarian cancer. The goal of surgery is to help stage the disease because this helps treatment decisions to be made, and to remove as much of the tumour as possible because this helps increase the chances of survival (Martin 2002). The staging system used is that of the International Federation of Gynaecology and Obstetrics.

After staging of the disease, patients may not have to receive any further treatment, although some may receive chemotherapy. Despite treatments, the disease recurs after primary therapy in 80% of women (Martin 2002).

Endometrial cancer

Cancer of the uterus, also known as 'womb cancer', is a fairly common type of cancer. It is the fifth most common cancer in women in the UK, with over 5200 new cases diagnosed each year (Cancer Research UK 2004). Endometrial cancer is rare in child-bearing years and the chance of developing it increases with age, as with most cancers occurring in women after the menopause (Porter 2002).

Anatomy and physiology

The uterus (womb) is a hollow pear-shaped organ. It is found between the bladder and rectum in a woman's pelvis. Most cancers of the uterus develop from cells lining its inner surface – the endometrium (Cancer Research UK 2004).

Risk factors

The primary risk factors for endometrial cancer are those that create an environment where the endometrium experiences prolonged or unopposed stimulation by oestrogen. Where women had received hormone replacement therapy (HRT) that was oestrogen-only therapy, the incidence of endometrial cancer increased. When this type of HRT was changed to both oestrogen and progesterone, the incidence of endometrial cancer decreased (Porter 2002).

Being overweight can also increase the risk of endometrial cancer, possibly because surplus fat will produce more oestrogen. Women who have never been pregnant are more likely to develop endometrial cancer than women with children and women who go through their menopause after the age of 52 may have an increased risk.

There is an increased risk of endometrial cancer for women who are being treated with tamoxifen for breast cancer. However, these cancers tend to be lower grade and lower stage. The incidence of endometrial cancer caused solely by tamoxifen use is difficult to determine because women with breast cancer are already at a higher risk for developing endometrial cancer (Porter 2002). According to Cancer Research UK (2004), the proven benefits of taking tamoxifen far outweigh the risk of developing endometrial cancer.

Prevention

Avoiding the use of oestrogen therapy on its own (unopposed oestrogen) is one strategy used in the prevention of endometrial cancer. HRT for the postmenopausal woman who still has a uterus now includes progesterone to prevent endometrial hyperplasia (Porter 2002). Emphasis on eating a healthy diet is also important. Women who eat low-fat or vegetarian diets have lower levels of oestrogen and oestradiol (female hormones) circulating in their plasma. Eating sensibly can also help prevent obesity, which is a risk factor for endometrial cancer (Brinton and Hoover 2000).

Screening

There is no early screening for endometrial cancer.

Signs and symptoms

The symptoms of endometrial cancer include:

- bleeding from the vagina after the menopause
- abnormal vaginal bleeding, which could be 'spotting' or very heavy around the time of the menopause or before
- pain in the pelvis, back or legs
- a change from the usual bowel habit
- weight loss
- difficult or painful urination (passing water).

These signs and symptoms may indicate endometrial cancer; however, they could indicate problems other than cancer. Endometrial cancer is often found in an early stage because the most common sign, vaginal bleeding, causes a woman to seek medical help (Porter 2002).

Diagnosis

Endometrial sampling is an essential step in diagnosis. Samples of the endometrium and cervical canal are taken. A pelvic examination ('internal') is performed to determine the size of the uterus and cervix and to see whether spread outside the uterus has occurred (Porter 2002, Cancer Research UK 2004). Since 1988 endometrial cancer has been surgically staged (Porter 2002) as follows:

- Stage I: endometrial cancer involves the uterus
- Stage II: involves the cervix
- Stage III: involves regional or distant spread to other organs

The grade of tumour and whether the cancer has spread outside the uterus are important for determination of the prognosis.

Treatment

A hysterectomy (removal of the uterus) and bilateral salpingo-oophorectomy (removal of both fallopian tubes and ovaries) are standard treatment. Removal of the lymph nodes may be performed to stage the cancer. In some women, the cancer is inoperable and in these cases the women would be offered primary radiotherapy (DiSaia and Creasman 2002). After clinical staging of the cancer, some women may be offered radiotherapy and chemotherapy, although most women with endometrial cancer are cured with surgery alone (Porter 2002).

Psychosocial issues

Patients with cancer may experience a range of emotions, including fright, guilt, frustration, helplessness, anger and denial (Jefferies 2002). Patients with cervical cancer might also feel upset with society's misconceptions that their disease is linked to promiscuity (Jefferies 2002). Women can also feel guilty if they feel that their disease is a result of their past sexual behaviour (Tabano et al. 2002). Removal of the uterus can alter a woman's self-image and perceived femininity. The uterus is a symbol of reproduction and, without it and the associated menstruation, a woman might feel that she is no longer a sexual being and that she has lost something that makes her female (Walsgrove 2001). The removal of the ovaries will cause menopausal symptoms of hot flushes, night sweats and mood swings; the patient may associate these with premature ageing and also equate her loss with diminished femininity and sexual attractiveness (Shell 1990).

The loss of fertility or sexual changes can be very traumatic for some women (Fischer 2002). All these changes can have a serious impact on quality of life.

The role of the nurse

Nurses have an important role to play, not only with women who have gynaecological cancers but also with healthy women. They should educate women about the screening procedures available to them and encourage them to attend for regular cervical smears. They could also educate women about what the signs and symptoms are of the cancers, so that they are aware of what is a normal change associated with ageing and what is abnormal. Women should be informed that any uterine bleeding in the postmenopausal period should have investigations. Advice on diet may be appropriate to help reduce the incidence of obesity, which is implicated in some cancers.

The nurse should design care by focusing on what is most important to these women through study of their experiences. Different people have different experiences (Fitch et al. 2001). Ovarian cancer affects sexual functioning and communication with patients about sexual issues is an important component of nursing care. Yet, in a small study of women with ovarian cancer, no patient received any written information and only two received brief verbal information about sexual issues (Stead et al. 2001). Nursing care needs to be comprehensive and to include both physical and psychosocial assessment.

Conclusion

Gynaecological cancers are not the most common cancers in women; however, they do carry a heavy physical and emotional burden (Tabano et al. 2002). Women may have to undergo surgery, radiotherapy and/or chemotherapy, and these treatments can affect a woman's quality of life. Common side effects of treatment, such as fatigue, anaemia, nausea and vomiting, can have a negative effect on the quality of life, and the loss of fertility, physical disfigurement and sexual changes can be traumatic for some women. Nurses have an important role to play by ensuring that they are aware of current social policy in relation to screening for gynaecological cancers and can inform women about screening available to them and the benefits of such screening. They can also help women by giving them up-to-date written information. The nurse should ensure that the physical, psychosocial and sexual needs of women are identified and attempts made to meet these needs.

References

Akhmedkhanov A, Toniolo P, Zeleniuch-Jacquotte A (2001) Aspirin and epithelial ovarian cancer. Prev Med 33: 682–7.

Anderson B, Lutgendorf S (1997) Quality of life in gynaecologic cancer survivors. CA Cancer J Clin 47: 218–25.

Anderson MC, Coulter CAE, Mason WP, Soutter WP (1997) Malignant disease of the cervix. In: Shaw R, Soutter WP, Stanton S (eds), Gynaecology. London: Churchill Livingstone.

Bicheno S (2004) Ovarian cancer. Cancer Nurs Pract 3(6): 12–15.

Blake P, Lambert H, Crawford R (1998) Gynaecological Oncology: A guide to clinical management. Oxford: Oxford University Press.

Bowes DE, Butler LJ (2002) Women living with ovarian cancer: dealing with an early death. Health Care Women Int 23: 135–48.
Brinton LA, Hoover RN (2000) Epidemiology of gynaecologic cancers. In: Hoskins WJ, Perez CA, Young RC (eds), Principles and Practice of Gynaecologic Oncology, 3rd edn. Philadelphia, PA: Lippincott, Williams & Wilkins, pp. 3–27.
Butcher M (2001) Education for women undergoing HPV testing. Prof Nurse 16: 1044–7.
Cancer Research UK (2004) Cervical Cancer online: www.cancerresearchuk.org/aboutcancer/specificcancers (last accessed 8/7/04).
Cherry C, Vacchiano J (2002) Ovarian cancer screening and protection. Semin Oncol Nurs 18: 167–73.
Claus EB, Schildkraut JM, Thompson WD, Douglas-Risch Neil J (1996) The genetic attributable risk of breast and ovarian cancer. Cancer 77: 2318–24.
Department of Health (2000) The NHS Cancer Plan: A plan for investment, a plan for reform. London: HMSO.
DiSaia PJ, Creasman WT (2002) Clinical Gynaecologic Oncology, 6th edn. St Louis, MO: Mosby.
Fischer M (2002) Cancer of the cervix. Semin Oncol Nurs 18: 193–9.
Fitch MI, Gray RE, Franssen E (2001) Perspectives on living with ovarian cancer: older women's views. Oncol Nurs Forum 24: 1433–42.
Goff BA, Mandel L, Muntz HG, Howard G, Melancon CH (2000) Ovarian cancer diagnosis. Results of a national ovarian cancer survey. Cancer 89: 2068–75.
Janicek MR, Averette HE (2001) Cervical cancer: prevention, diagnosis, and therapeutics. CA Cancer J Clin 51: 92–114.
Jeffries H (2002) The psychosocial care of a patient with cervical cancer. Cancer Nurs Pract 1 (5): 19–25.
Jolley S (2004) Quality in colposcopy. Nurs Stand 18(23): 39–44.
Lamb M, Moore M (1997) Invasive cancer of the cervix. In: Moore G (ed.), Women and Cancer: A gynaecologic oncology nursing perspective. Sudbury, MA: Jones & Bartlett.
Martin VR (2000) Ovarian cancer. In: Yarbro CH, Frogge MH, Goodman M, Groenwald SL (eds), Cancer Nursing Principles and Practice, 5th edn. Sudbury, MA: Jones & Bartlett, pp. 1374–99.
Martin VR (2002) Ovarian cancer. Semin Oncol Nurs 18: 174–83.
Moore-Higgs GL (ed.) (2000) Women and Cancer: A gynaecologic oncology nursing perspective, 2nd edn. Sudbury, MA: Jones & Bartlett.
NHS Cervical Screening Programme (2000) Reducing the Risk. Sheffield: NHSCSP.
Porter S (2002) Endometrial cancer. Semin Oncol Nurs 18: 200–6.
Rako S (1996) The Hormone of Desire: The truth about sexuality, menopause and testosterone. New York: Harmony Books.
Royal College of Nursing (1999) Gynaecological Cancer Information and Guidance for Nurses. London: RCN.
Shell (1990) Sexuality for patients with gynaecologic cancer. Clinical Issues for Perineal Women's Health Nurses 1: 479–514.
Stead ML, Fallowfield L, Brown JM, Selby P (2001) Communication about sexual problems and sexual concerns in ovarian cancer: Qualitative study. BMJ 323: 836–7.
Tabano M, Condosta D, Coons M (2002) Symptoms affecting quality of life in women with gynaecologic cancer. Semin Oncol Nurs 18: 223–30.
Walsgrove H (2001) Hysterectomy. Nurs Stand 15(29): 47–53.

Chapter 8

Treatments for cancer

Treatments for cancer are based on a combination of experience, expertise and research. Multidisciplinary teamwork and effective treatment planning are necessary in order to select the most effective treatment for an individual. Different combinations of treatments are more likely to control the spread of cancer and include, in the main, surgery, radiotherapy and chemotherapy. Knowledge of the biological basis of cancer has had an impact on how these treatments are used, both independently and in combination (Corner and Bailey 2001). Evidence suggests that treatment, however difficult, is accepted by most cancer sufferers, even when it may offer only a slim chance of cure. Heavy investment in the development of these treatments has left little resources for the management of actual and potential harmful side effects and, for some, letting go of treatment becomes very difficult, even when all hope of containing the disease has passed (Yarbro et al. 2000, Corner and Bailey 2001).

Surgery

Surgery is one of the most important treatment options for solid tumours and has remained so despite advances in our knowledge of the pattern of spread of the disease. Surgery is the oldest form of cancer treatment available, particularly for those with solid tumours: 60% of cancer patients will undergo some form of surgery (Foulds 2002). Advances in surgery itself have allowed for more complex and radical surgery, with the help of increasing knowledge of the use of antibiotics, advanced technology in critical care and improvements in the use of prosthetics after radical surgery (Nevidjon and Sowers 2000, Corner and Bailey 2001, Foulds 2002).

For surgery to be effective all cancer cells should be removed so surgery must involve the resection of the entire tumour mass with a safe margin of normal tissue around it. Several factors influence surgical treatment decisions:

- Cancer growth rate: slow growing cancers are more likely to be contained in the local area and are less likely to have spread.

- Metastatic potential: some cancers rarely spread and have the potential to be cured with surgery; if spread is to local areas a cure might still be achieved. Where cancers have spread to distant sites, surgery might be avoided or used to control local spread.
- Cancer histology: surgery is suitable only for solid cancers and relies on the position of the cancer, e.g. whether it is near vital structures or the cancer is deeply embedded in its local area.
- Patient's quality of life: the severity of the patient's physical condition needs to be taken into account when making surgical treatment decisions. Risks and benefits need to be carefully balanced and should be acceptable to the patient (Corner and Bailey 2001, Foulds 2002).

Definitive surgical interventions are used as part of the treatment process but surgery is not limited to treatment alone and can include prevention, diagnosis and staging, reconstruction and palliation.

Definitive surgery

The goal of definitive surgery is to remove as much of the cancer as possible with a margin of disease-free tissue surrounding it. One of the aims of surgery should be tissue and function preservation. Cryosurgery and laser surgery are used for skin, cervical and prostate cancer. Local resections are carried out for small cancers: the whole cancer is removed along with a clear margin. For larger cancers with further spread, surgery is more radical with removal of local and regional tissue as well as the primary cancer. It must be remembered that surgery is a localized treatment and is often used in combination with other treatments to produce an optimal effect. Surgery, as has been stated, is the primary treatment; all other treatments are adjuvant or extra. Adjuvant treatments can be given at different stages, e.g. preoperatively usually termed 'neoadjuvant', postoperatively or adjuvant, and sometimes intraoperatively.

Definitive surgery also has a role in the resection of metastatic disease where cure is thought possible. A single site of metastasis can be removed when the primary cancer is thought to have been eradicated. Successful surgical resection for metastatic disease can take place in the lung, liver and brain (Corner and Bailey 2001, Foulds 2002).

Diagnostic surgery

Diagnostic techniques are now so improved and refined that most cancer patients should not need traditional surgery to diagnose disease; other less invasive methods are available.

Biopsies

- Fine needle aspiration: the use of a needle and syringe to aspirate cells. This procedure is quick and well tolerated and can be used along with computed tomography (CT) or ultrasonography when the cancer cannot be seen or palpated (e.g. in screen-detected breast cancers).
- Needle core biopsy: a larger-bore needle is used along with some instrumentation to collect tissue; a local anaesthetic is used for this procedure.
- Incisional biopsy: a wedge of tissue is removed from a larger cancer mass.
- Excisional biopsy: excision of the entire cancer for diagnostic purposes; it can also be the definitive surgery if there are clear margins of disease-free tissue.

Endoscopies

Endoscopies are used to access and view lumina with the advantage of taking a biopsy at the same time if necessary. Flexible endoscopic instruments make the procedure more tolerable for the patient, although mild sedation is often necessary. Different types of endoscopy include: bronchoscopy for the lungs, gastroscopy for the stomach and colonoscopy for the bowel.

Examination under anaesthetic

This is occasionally used for examination or biopsy if the suspected cancer is inaccessible.

Laparotomy

This was historically used to diagnose gastrointestinal and gynaecological cancers before the advent of superior diagnostic and imaging tools.

Prophylactic surgery

Prophylactic surgery is preventive and is aimed at individuals with a family history of a specific type of cancer. The surgery removes non-vital tissue affected by different types of cancer and, in doing so, can lower the risk from the disease. Examples include mastectomy for familial breast cancer, oophorectomy for familial ovarian cancer and colectomy for hereditary non-polyposis colorectal cancer.

Reconstructive surgery

Recent developments in surgery have allowed surgeons to repair anatomical defects and improve function and cosmesis. Reconstructive surgery can be offered in some instances at the same time as definitive surgery. Reconstructive surgery can facilitate self-esteem and lifestyle and help the patient cope with diagnosis and treatment (Corner and Bailey 2001). A simple reconstruction might involve a skin graft after excision of a skin cancer. A more complicated reconstruction might be the reconstruction of the tongue with a graft from the forearm. It is important to remember, however, that, although great advances have been made with surgical techniques, the reconstructed area will not be the same as the original, so a balance between optimism and realism is necessary.

Palliative surgery

The main goal of palliative surgery is to relieve suffering and minimize the symptoms of the disease; it should not be undertaken where there is a risk of morbidity or mortality or if quality of life will not be improved. For some cancers, the line between definitive or curative surgery and palliative surgery is a fine one. Sometimes palliative surgery is essential, e.g. to relieve bowel obstruction and when a cancer is causing pressure on vital organs or blood vessels. Palliative surgery is very individual and based on the needs of the patient on a day-to-day basis.

Nursing care

Current understanding of cancer biology and the natural history of cancer has caused the role of surgery to be questioned and modified, particularly in the case of radical surgery (Foulds 2002). Although this approach is still valid for some types of cancer, for others, e.g. breast cancer, a less radical approach can achieve adequate control and survival.

When looking after the patient undergoing surgery or cancer, it is important to remember the holistic nature of care. For the cancer patient every aspect of the cancer journey is set within a unique set of life experiences. For some patients there might be optimism and for others fear. Patients require support from the multidisciplinary team, working together collaboratively to provide holistic care for the patient and family (Nevidjon and Sowers 2000, Corner and Bailey 2001, Foulds 2002). The general principles of surgical care should apply, with the patient in optimal biopsychosocial condition for surgery. In almost all cases the patient should know which surgical procedure they are having. This, together with good general preparation, should allow the patient to begin postoperative recovery with reduced anxiety. Postoperatively special attention should be taken with anxiety and pain management, wound care, nutritional support and emotional care.

Chemotherapy

Chemotherapy involves the systemic administration of chemical agents to eradicate or control the growth of cancer. The term 'chemotherapy' was originally used at the beginning of the twentieth century to refer to the use of substances with specific toxicity towards micro-organisms such as bacteria. When used in cancer treatment, the aim of the chemical agents is to disrupt cellular replication by inhibiting the synthesis of new genetic material or by causing irreparable damage to the cellular DNA (Corner and Bailey 2001, Morgan 2003). Chemotherapy in cancer care can be curative when all cancer cells are destroyed; it can be used to control the disease by preventing further cancer growth and palliatively to reduce the impact of tumour load and thereby manage symptoms such as pain or breathlessness (Corner and Bailey 2001). Hodgkin's disease, childhood lymphoblastic leukaemia and some testicular cancers can be cured with chemotherapy.

Chemotherapy and surgery combined can offer the potential for a cure in breast and colorectal cancer. Chemotherapy in small cell lung cancers can offer increased survival (Morgan 2003). Chemotherapy can be used as the main treatment modality and is referred to as definitive chemotherapy but it is used more commonly to support primary surgical treatment. Adjuvant chemotherapy is used after surgery to eradicate any micrometastatic disease. Neoadjuvant chemotherapy is used before surgery to reduce the size of the cancer and maximize the effectiveness of further treatments. When using chemotherapy key definitions are used in relation to the response of the disease:

- CR: complete response (disappearance of all disease)
- PR: partial response (50% decrease in disease)
- NC: no change (no decrease beyond 50%, no increase beyond 25%)
- PD: progressive disease (an increase of more than 25%).

Chemotherapy and the cell cycle

Chemotherapeutic drugs work by killing cancerous cells during specific phases of their reproductive cycle; however, they also destroy healthy cells. The aim of chemotherapy is to find a dose strength and duration that will kill cancerous cells but allow normal cells, which have the ability to repair themselves, to survive.

Chemotherapeutic drugs are divided into two main classes: cell cycle specific and cell cycle non-specific. Those agents that are non-specific can act on several or all cell cycle phases; cell cycle-specific agents act only on a particular phase of the cell cycle. Cell cycle-non-specific agents act on the basis that the greater the dose given the greater the number of cancer cells that are killed. Cell cycle-non-specific drugs are usually given as a single injection. Cell cycle-specific drugs do not act in the same way and their effect is limited and not related to dosage. Cell cycle-specific drugs are usually administered as a continuous infusion.

When chemotherapy is administered, only a fraction of cancer cells is destroyed and subsequent cycles of chemotherapy are necessary to reduce the total number of cancer cells. Cell cycle-specific and cell cycle non-specific chemotherapeutic agents can be used in combination to destroy the maximum amount of cancer cells. When the number of cancer cells reduces, the body's natural defence mechanisms can play a part in destroying the remaining cancer cells (Corner and Bailey 2001, Morgan 2003).

Chemotherapy side effects

Chemotherapeutic drugs affect healthy cells as well as cancer cells and particularly those cells that are rapidly dividing and in a constant state of cell division, such as hair follicle cells, bone marrow cells and those cells lining the gut. The effect on the patient can be devastating and can add to the already monumental problems being faced:

- Hair follicle cells: hair loss
- The gut: nausea and vomiting
- Bone marrow: increased susceptibility to infection, anaemia and clotting problems caused by bone marrow suppression and its effect on white and red blood cells and platelets.

Administration of chemotherapy

The administration of chemotherapeutic agents takes into account the effect of the drug on the cell cycle and the effect on healthy cells:

- Continuous infusional chemotherapy: effective when tumour cells are in a specific phase of the cell cycle, the anti-cancer agent is present when the sensitive phase of the cycle is reached.
- Intermittent chemotherapy: intervals allow for the recovery of normal cells.
- Combination chemotherapy: different drugs have different actions on the cell; use of a combination of drugs reduces the likelihood of resistance.
- High-dose chemotherapy: this can cause toxicity in bone marrow and can be used if bone marrow (or stem cells) is first taken from the patient and returned at a later date, usually 48–96 h after chemotherapy has been administered.

The effect of the chemotherapy on the individual and where and when the chemotherapy is administered are also taken into account and depend on several factors:

- The patient's age and general health
- The planned drug regimen and method of administration
- Any additional therapy, e.g. hydration
- The need to correct deficits, e.g. nutritional support
- Anticipated severity of side effects
- The wishes of the patient and the family.

There are several routes of administration for chemotherapeutic drugs mainly determined by the type of drug and the effect that it exerts:

- Intra-arterial: chemotherapy is injected directly into the blood supply of the tumour; this route reduces side effects caused by low concentrations of chemotherapy elsewhere in the body. This method can be used to treat several cancers.
- Intrapleural: chemotherapy is inserted between the pleura which line the lung. This treatment is used for pleural effusion (the pleural cavity becomes filled with fluid) which can occur with several different cancers.
- Intravesical: direct instillation of chemotherapy into the bladder for bladder cancer.
- Intrathecal: chemotherapy injected directly into the cerebrospinal fluid (CSF) of the spinal cord via a lumbar puncture.
- Intraventricular: chemotherapy injected directly into the CSF of the brain.
- Intraperitoneal: direct instillation of drugs into the peritoneal cavity, the peritoneum being the lining of the abdominal cavity.
- Topical: a cream applied to cancers of the skin.
- Oral: many chemotherapeutic drugs are taken by mouth and then absorbed by the gut.
- Intramuscular: direct injection of chemotherapeutic drugs into the muscle.
- Subcutaneous: direct injection into the subcutaneous tissue; this route is not used often as a result of the irritant nature of the drugs being used so close to the surface of the skin.

- Intravenous: the most common route of administration of chemotherapeutic drugs, directly into the vein.
- Central venous access: several different devices are available that allow long-term venous access. The devices are skin tunnelled in order to stabilize the catheter and create an additional barrier, minimizing the potential for infection. The patient's subcutaneous tissue grows in and around the cuff of the catheter in the skin tunnel before it reaches its point of entry into the vein (Gabriel 2003):
  - PICCs (peripherally inserted central catheters) – threaded through the veins of the arm at the antecubital fossa into the superior vena cava
  - skin tunnelled catheter, e.g. a Hickman line, with single, double or triple lumina; entry to the vena cava through veins in the neck area (usually subclavian).
  - implantable port – the PICC and Hickman line are visible where they exit the skin, chemotherapy being introduced externally; the implantable port lies just under the skin of the chest wall, offering hidden access to a single lumen (Gabriel 2003).
- Infusional ambulatory chemotherapy: refers to chemotherapy administered at home. A number of chemotherapeutic drugs maintain concentration in the blood when given by continuous infusion. The effect of the continuous infusion is beneficial for those tumours with a slow cell cycle, where the effect can be measured in days rather than hours. The toxicity of the chemotherapy can also be reduced if given in smaller doses over a longer time period. The effectiveness of this form of treatment can be measured financially in the reduction of costs related to hospitalization. The real benefit, however, can be to patients and their families, who are enabled to care for themselves within their own environment. This can be measured in terms of less psychosocial distress and reduced risk of cross-infection while immunocompromised. Ambulatory chemotherapy is not suitable for all patients and should be decided on an individual holistic basis, taking into account all the safety issues involved for the staff as well as the patient.

Nursing care

The main areas of care relating to chemotherapy include: health and safety issues with regard to the safe handling and administration of chemotherapeutic agents; care of the site of access; psychosocial issues related to this stage of treatment; and care related to the side effects of chemotherapy. The last two issues are discussed in later chapters. Chemotherapy should be administered only by health-care professionals who have appropriate expertise and experience in caring for cancer patients and administering chemotherapy.

Health and safety

The Health and Safety at Work Act 1974 and Control of Substances Hazardous to Health (COSHH) regulations offer guidelines on preparation, handling and management of spillage of chemotherapeutic agents. These drugs are known to induce genetic mutations, produce physical defects in a foetus and induce cancer development. Some studies have shown these effects in hospital staff working with chemotherapeutic drugs. Where safety policies are adhered to, the risk can be reduced or removed. One of the key areas for safety is the use of protective clothing; depending on the drugs being used, this might be an apron and gloves but might include an overall, non-absorbent armlets, eye protection and a facemask. The procedure should be fully explained to the patient, as well as the rationale for wearing the protective clothing. The emotional distress experienced by the patient can easily be exacerbated by being approached by someone who looks like they are wearing armour. Good communication is paramount to put patients at ease and make them feel comfortable within a therapeutic environment where they may be for a period of days or weeks (Corner and Bailey 2001, Morgan 2003, Roberts 2003).

Care of access site

As has been highlighted, chemotherapeutic drugs are extremely toxic. Some drugs have vesicant properties, which means that they are highly caustic to veins and soft tissue. When administering these drugs directly into the vein or into a central venous access site, some of the drug may escape from the vein. This extravasation allows the drug to infiltrate the skin and surrounding tissues, causing damage, necrosis or tissue death. The patient may complain of pain and a burning sensation at the site; the site may also be reddened and swollen. The incidence of extravasation is lower among experienced nurses in specialist units compared with nurses in general areas (Del Gaudio and Menonna-Quinn 1998, Corner and Bailey 2001).

Radiotherapy

Radiotherapy is a treatment used for local as opposed to systemic management of cancer. Over 50% of patients with cancer will receive radiotherapy at some time on their cancer pathway. Radiotherapy can be offered as adjuvant and neoadjuvant treatment, as curative treatment and in palliation. Its success depends on the sensitivity of the cancer to radiation as well as the tolerance of the surrounding tissues.

Radiotherapy uses ionizing radiation to damage cellular DNA and cause cell death; unfortunately as with chemotherapy both normal and cancerous cells are affected.

Ionizing radiation

Ionizing radiation produces ionization of atoms and molecules; it causes atoms of cells in its path to lose orbiting electrons. When electrons are released from their orbit, energy in the form of free electrons is released at high speed and dislodges more electrons from neighbouring atoms, which in turn release energy. The electrically charged particles are called ions and their process of development is called ionization. Ionization is responsible for the chemical and biological changes that occur to tissues. This process can be visualized by thinking about marbles! When one marble knocks others in its path, it causes them to scatter, creating more movement in a cascade (Yarbro et al. 2000, Corner and Bailey 2001).

Radiobiology

Radiotherapy damages DNA and causes single- or double-strand breaks in its structure; this damage may be repairable. Normal cells have a greater ability to repair themselves than cancer cells. Differences in effectiveness of radiotherapy are determined by:

- individual cancer cell response
- the presence of oxygen
- the number of cells actively dividing
- the rate of growth of the cancerous cells.

The cell cycle is most sensitive to radiation during mitosis and the G2 phase, with the greatest resistance during DNA synthesis (Nevidjon and Sowers 2000).

Treatment

The dose of radiation is described as the amount of energy absorbed per unit mass of tissue. This is measured in grays (Gy): 1 gray = 1 joule/kg. For a curative course of radiotherapy the dose ranges from 55 to 65 Gy and is given in daily treatments of 1.6–2.5 Gy over 4–6 weeks. This break down of treatment into limited doses over a long time period is known as fractionation (Nevidjon and Sowers 2000, Corner and Bailey 2001). Delivery can be by the following methods:

- External beam radiotherapy: this form of radiotherapy uses a beam at a defined distance away from the patient. A linear accelerator delivers the radiotherapy in the form of high-energy X-rays at some distance from the skin surface (known as skin sparing, to prevent skin damage).
- Brachytherapy: this involves the delivery of radiation directly to the cancer by placing the source of the radiation in direct contact with the cancer. The cancer then receives a high dose of radiation with little escaping to the surrounding tissues.
- Oral or by injection: radioactive isotopes can be administered to target tissues where the isotopes are known to concentrate.

Side effects

The side effects of radiotherapy develop in several stages: acute side effects usually resolve in time but late stage side effects may take years to develop and can be progressive and chronic. Research and clinical trials are attempting to address the issue of radiosensitivity, in an effort to determine who is at most risk and whether problems will be late or early stage. Radiosensitivity is often related to total dose of radiation and sensitivity of particular tissues; however, there are many exceptions. Research is beginning to show that there is a genetic predisposition to hypersensitivity. The main side effects from radiotherapy affect the skin and the gut and can cause fatigue; the last two side effects are discussed in Chapter 10.

Skin reactions

Modern 'skin-sparing' radiotherapy techniques have reduced the incidence of skin reactions to radiotherapy; however, this is still the largest area in which nurses are asked to intervene. Erythema (reddening of skin) and moist desquamation (outer layer of skin removed by scaling) are the most common effects and often leave patients feeling that they have been 'burnt' by their therapy. The average time for repopulation of skin cells is 4 weeks; repopulation is hampered by continuing treatment, particularly when it does not keep up with skin loss. Factors influencing skin vulnerability include: the site of radiotherapy if skin folds and creases are involved or if the area is susceptible to friction; recent surgery at the site of radiotherapy; diabetes or vascular disease; and the use of irritant skin care products. Management of radiotherapy-related skin problems remain diverse and research in this area falls behind research into conventional wound management. The effect on the patient can be extreme, influencing body image and sexuality, limiting function, and affecting activities of daily living including sleep disturbances. The key cornerstones of care include:

- promotion of patient comfort
- prevention of infection
- prevention of further skin damage.

They can be achieved in some way by keeping skin clean and dry and using moisturizing cream as necessary; this should always follow local protocols in the absence of general evidence-based guidelines. Clothes should be loose and cotton based and skin should be protected from the harmful rays of the sun.

Nursing care

Radiotherapy is usually organized as an outpatient treatment and, as a consequence, nursing support may not be available to patients accessing treatment. Some cancer centres have recognized this and have nurses or radiographers in specialist supportive roles. Supportive care can encompass information giving, counselling, social support and management of side effects, with the aim of reducing biopsychosocial problems associated with radiotherapy. There is still a lack of consistency in radiotherapy treatment strategies, management of side effects and supportive strategies. The National Institute for Clinical Effectiveness guidelines (NICE 2004) *Improving Supportive and Palliative Care for Adults with Cancer* emphasise the importance of partnership working with patients and their families with a service that is holistic and responsive to patients' needs.

Radiotherapy treatment can sometimes last several weeks, starting with the initial planning stage, treatment phase and post-treatment phase. The importance of supportive care cannot be overemphasized. Excellent communication skills and the ability to impart clear information will help the patient and the family gain an understanding of the procedures involved and the possible side effects of treatment. Previously reported patient anxiety has focused on patients not understanding their treatment and the procedures involved, and a lack of orientation to a radiotherapy unit that is often separate from other facilities. Time taken to orient patients to their surroundings, explaining length of time of treatment and providing information on car parking and refreshment areas will serve to reduce anxiety and promote an optimal therapeutic relationship. Supportive care in radiotherapy should also address 'separation anxiety', which is often felt by patients when treatment finishes. The routine of several weeks of treatment can afford some stability to lives shattered by a cancer diagnosis and the loss of that stability should be recognized and discussed before completion of treatment so that support measures can put in place if necessary (Nevidjon and Sowers 2000, Yarbro et al. 2000, Corner and Bailey 2001).

Endocrine therapies

Cancers arising in organs that are influenced by hormones are amenable to hormonal treatment, e.g. the breast, prostate, thyroid and uterus. Hormones are produced by endocrine glands; they circulate and control different functions in the body.

Endocrine therapy is not usually looked upon as curative but can be used as adjuvant and neoadjuvant treatment to encourage disease regression as well as for disease prevention. Some cells are sensitive to hormone deprivation and die, whereas others are not sensitive and continue to grow and spread (Corner and Bailey 2001).

The effectiveness of endocrine therapy varies according to the type of cancer; in breast cancer the chance of achieving a response lies between 30 and 40%; in prostate cancer this rises to 80% (Nevidjon and Sowers 2000, Corner and Bailey 2001).

The effectiveness of hormone therapy in controlling disease needs to be balanced against the possibility of severe side effects. Sometimes the side effects can be of such magnitude that the quality of life of the patient is markedly reduced, e.g. in breast cancer hormone treatments can cause severe menopausal symptoms: weight gain, hot sweats and vaginal dryness. These effects can have a marked effect on body image and sexuality as well as general quality of life, further impacting on the effects of the disease process and other treatment modalities (Corner and Bailey 2001).

Biotherapy and gene therapy

Biotherapy is the use of biological sources or agents that affect the body's biological responses to cancer, in particular the use of the immune system. The purpose of the immune system is to recognize, destroy and clear foreign bodies. The body recognizes cancer as being a foreign body and elicits an immune response in an attempt to destroy it, as it does with any bacterium that enters the body. Biotherapy uses the principles of immunity in an attempt to destroy cancer cells, e.g. serotherapy uses antibodies created in the lab that recognize and bind to particular cancers. Some biotherapy treatments have been shown to be successful, when used together with other treatments; others have resulted in failure. Clinicians and scientists alike look on biotherapy as the fourth treatment modality after surgery, radiotherapy and chemotherapy, and continue to support research in this area (Nevidjon and Sowers 2000).

Gene therapy is a new and rapidly evolving area that has clinical implications in the treatment of heart disease, arthritis and neurodegenerative conditions, as well as cancer. It can be defined as a treatment aimed at destroying cancers by correcting genetic defects, manipulating genes or both. Like biotherapy, gene therapy has the potential to modify the body's biological response by genetic manipulation (Nevidjon and Sowers 2000, Chester 2002). Gene therapy is used in two ways:

1. To add a new function to cells: this can be to correct a genetic error or to add a function.
2. To label a cell for future identification by gene marking (Chester 2002).

Gene therapy is still in early development. The main role of the nurse is to provide information and education on the different treatment options available and to support the patient.

Conclusion

Different combinations of treatments are more likely to control the spread of cancer. In the main treatments include surgery, chemotherapy and radiotherapy. As has been stated, multidisciplinary teamwork and treatment planning are necessary in order to select the most effective treatment plan for an individual. Health-care professionals must work closely with patients and their families, particularly when patients are offered a choice of treatments. Excellent communication skills and the giving of clear information will empower patients, enabling them to work with the multidisciplinary team to select an appropriate treatment plan.

References

Chester M (2002) The role of the gene therapy nurse in cancer care. Cancer Nurs Pract 1(8): 25–9.

Corner J, Bailey C (eds) (2001) Cancer Nursing: Care in context. London: Blackwell.
Del Gaudio D, Menonna-Quinn D (1998) Chemotherapy: potential occupational hazards. Am J Nurs 98(11): 59–65 (http://nursingcenter.com).
Foulds E (2002) Surgical oncology. Cancer Nurs Pract 1(2): 33–8.
Gabriel J (2003) Peripherally inserted central catheters: patient involvement. Cancer Nurs Pract 2(8): 27–31.
Morgan G (2003) Chemotherapy and the cell cycle. Cancer Nurs Pract 2(1): 27–30.
National Institute for Clinical Effectiveness (2004) Improving Supportive and Palliative Care for Adults with Cancer. London: NICE.
Nevidjon B, Sowers K (eds) (2000) A Nurse's Guide to Cancer Care. Philadelphia, PA: Lippincott.
Roberts R (2003) Reducing the risks. Cancer Nurs Pract 2(4): 22–3
Yarbro CH, Frogge MH, Goodman M, Groenwald SL (eds) (2000) Cancer Nursing Principles and Practice, 5th edn. London: Jones & Bartlett.

Chapter 9

Complementary therapies

Complementary therapies are defined as those therapies that are taken together with conventional medicine (Hann et al. 2003). Complementary therapies are no longer an obscure issue in health care but an adjunct to conventional treatment, practised by a wide variety of practitioners and used by a large number of patients. Complementary therapies purport to treat the widest range of physical and psychological illnesses. Alternative therapies usually refer to those therapies with unproven benefits: unorthodox, unconventional and questionable, and generally used in place of orthodox medical treatment. It should be remembered that many alternative therapies are only alternative to the west and in significant sections of the world it is western medicine that is alternative (Kinghorn and Gamlin 2001).

In the UK, traditional medicine is dominant and is used to treat cancer, with most people seeking an alternative only when conventional approaches have failed. However, in recent years the number of patients who engage in some form of complementary therapy either during or after standard treatment has increased. Traditional barriers between traditional and alternative therapies are breaking down as society's perceptions and expectations of health care change, particularly in relation to perceived failings of traditional therapies including a lack of cancer cures (Kinghorn and Gamlin 2001, Farrant 2003, Hann et al. 2003).

Historically, the west has focused on the study of medicine and the effect of disease on the body and its functions. Spiritual and mental function such as consciousness, creativity, emotions, beliefs, subjectivity, thoughts, feelings and experience were largely excluded. For centuries the mind and spirit as causative factors in illness have been ignored; however, psychological, emotional and spiritual links are now being rigorously investigated (Kinghorn and Gamlin 2001).

Modern ethical thinking respects patient autonomy and empowerment, the growth in complementary therapies reflecting social and political changes that have influenced the relationship between health care and the patient. According to Kinghorn and Gamlin (2001) the patient takes far more responsibility towards feeling well, has a redefined relationship with nature and actively pursues preventive medicine. Stevenson (1996) suggests that it is important to remember that it is not claimed that complementary therapies will cure the disease, but that they offer support to enhance quality of life and provide symptom relief. Patients are encouraged to accept all appropriate forms of therapy including conventional surgery, radiotherapy and chemotherapy.

Interdisciplinary team working is essential throughout the treatment trajectory and particularly when complementary therapies are being used. It is estimated that only about half of cancer patients who use complementary therapies inform their doctor, which can be detrimental to the holistic care of the patient. Health-care professionals in cancer care should be familiar with the subject of complementary therapies and should be open to discussion with their patients. Working with colleagues from different disciplines can be challenging but also very rewarding. There is increasing evidence of effective collaboration between mainstream and complementary practitioners in a variety of settings. Much has been written about the need for mutual respect and honesty, open and flexible attitudes, a common purpose and a clear definition of roles. In those centres that combine both mainstream and complementary therapies, interdisciplinary teamworking is evolving rapidly (Peace and Simons 1996).

There are several advantages and disadvantages for the patient accessing complementary therapies.

Advantages

- Patient empowerment and a reduced sense of helplessness, particularly when using therapies such as guided imagery.
- Participation usually requires patient empowerment and reduced paternalism.
- The nature of complementary therapies generally allows the practitioner to afford more time to the patient.
- There is reduced pharmacological intervention for symptom control, particularly with the use of acupuncture for pain, relaxation for anxiety and aromatherapy for insomnia.
- There is heightened self-awareness, possibly as a result of the relaxing nature of therapies.
- There is immediate benefit, although this may be short term.

Disadvantages

- No therapy is completely safe and any intervention should be investigated.
- Some people prefer to be passive and enjoy paternalism in their treatment.
- Complementary therapies are time-consuming and expensive, and are perhaps an option only for those who can afford them when funding is not present.

- Arguments abound with regard to safety, efficacy and funding for complementary medicine, with the patient's perspective being the one to which the least attention is paid.

The government is monitoring those nurses delivering complementary therapies in order to provide patient protection. The Prince of Wales Foundation for Integrated Health has been given almost £1 million to devise voluntary methods of self-regulation for practitioners offering services such as homoeopathy, aromatherapy and reflexology, with each discipline having its own regulatory body.

The therapies

Surveys show that 30% of people living with cancer use complementary therapies mostly provided in hospices and hospitals, but with some outreach into the voluntary sector. The touch therapies such as aromatherapy, massage and reflexology are provided in over 90% of services with mind–body therapies such as visualization and relaxation being offered by 80% of service providers (Prince of Wales Foundation for Integrated Health and National Council for Hospice and Specialist Palliative Care or PWFIH and NCHSPC 2003).

Touch therapies

The best available evidence suggests that massage, aromatherapy and reflexology are useful in the following ways (PWFIH and NCHSPC 2003):

- To promote relaxation
- To alleviate anxiety
- To reduce depression
- To reduce pain
- To reduce nausea
- To alleviate symptoms such as breathlessness, constipation, diarrhoea, pain, nausea, fatigue and poor appetite
- To improve sleep patterns
- To reduce stress and tension
- To reduce psychological distress and provide emotional support
- To improve well-being and quality of life
- To live with an altered body image.

Aromatherapy

Aromatherapy or the use of essential oils to promote well-being and health and for cosmetic purposes has existed for thousands of years and is evidenced in the artefacts of the ancient Greeks and Egyptians. Essential oils from trees, bark, flowers and fruits are commonly used for massage and also for inhalation. Many plant species contain essential oils, highly fragrant and flammable essences that evaporate quickly. Aromatherapists in the UK are trained to use essential oils topically and through inhalation. Essential oils are applied in a variety of ways including:

- massage
- vaporizers
- baths
- creams
- lotions
- compresses.

The therapeutic effect of aromatherapy results from a combination of the physiological effects of the oils and the relaxation of massage. As the fragrance stimulates the senses hormones may be released that enhance mood (PWFIH and NCHSPC 2003).

In the UK aromatherapy was introduced by the beauty industry and was later combined with massage for stress management. Although many therapeutic uses for essential oils are recognized, the stress reduction properties of oils are powerfully advocated in palliative care (Kinghorn and Gamlin 2001). According to Kite et al. (1998) aromatherapy has a role at every stage in the cancer journey to alleviate stress, anxiety, fear and tension. They go on to suggest, however, that it is also time-consuming and expensive and does involve holistic care delivered by an interdisciplinary team.

Oncology and palliative care units are increasingly using complementary therapies, in particular aromatherapy massage. The aim of the therapy is to promote relaxation and ease tension by using essential oils to massage areas of the body. Evidence from patients suggests that this can improve physical symptoms, quality of life and mood (Wilcock et al. 2004).

Massage

Touch is as vital in illness as it is in health and can be described within two categories: touch incidental to general nursing activities and touch that is expressive or caring. Both forms of touch can hold difficulties for the nurse and patient, including misinterpretation of intent and meaning across culture and gender. Touch-based therapy can be useful when a clearly defined aim has been consented to such as acupressure for nausea, acupuncture for pain control and massage for insomnia. The experience of one health-care professional enhanced the care-giving experience:

> I have often felt humbled by the responses to some of the simple and time limited massages I have given, such as foot massage. Some of the most moving and emotional responses have been from the elderly who have possibly not been touched for many years. Their sense of joy and gratitude in receiving tender, respectful, appropriate and loving touch has reminded me that we remain sensual and sexual beings until we die. Others have responded with outpourings of grief as the part of their body most ravaged by surgery and radiotherapy has been touched. Opportunities are created for talking and the sharing of experiences, both painful and joyful.
>
> Macnish (2001, p. 105)

The time given to patients in this way may be as important and relevant to them as more orthodox treatments.

Research studies in massage for cancer patients suggest that massage either with or without an essential oil is beneficial in reducing levels of anxiety in patients and is an acceptable form of therapy. A short, slow-stroke back massage was shown to lower anxiety scores, heart rate and blood pressure when assessed over a 20-minute period (Wilkinson et al. 1999).

Many health-care professionals feel concern at offering the cancer patient massage in case the massage encourages the movement of cancer cells. Some oncologists have stated that there is no evidence to suggest that gentle massage increases the spread of cancerous cells and that cancer is not a contraindication to receiving gentle massage (PWFIH and NCHSPC 2003). Massage therapists are, however, advised to show caution over tumour sites because any mechanical force on a tumour exhibiting uncontrolled growth may influence spread. The importance of adequate training and regulation is key to practice in this area (PWFIH and NCHSPC 2003).

Reflexology

Reflexology is based on the principle that there are reflex areas in the feet and hands that correspond to all of the glands, organs and parts of the body, and the purpose of applying pressure to the reflex points in the feet is to release congestion, promote the flow of energy and promote well-being through the body's natural balance (PWFIH and NCHSPC 2003).

Reflexologists aim to feel areas that have an altered texture at specific points in the foot, indicating an imbalance, weakness or disease. Different types of foot treatment have been used in various cultures across the world since ancient times; however, in the west, reflexology developed in the twentieth century.

There is much anecdotal evidence supporting the use of reflexology in cancer care for relaxation, well-being and stress relief. Despite the lack of evidence, surveys, studies and investigations of patient use reveal that reflexology is one of the most widely used therapies in cancer care (Hodgson 2000, Hann et al. 2003, PWFIH and NCHSPC 2003).

Mind-body therapies

Relaxation and guided imagery

The central belief of relaxation and guided imagery is that what a person believes, thinks and feels affects every cell in the body. Imagery in thoughts, pictures, sounds, memories, feelings and sensations forms the basis of how the individuals experience their bodies, their relationships, work, the environment as well as their emotional and spiritual lives. In guided imagery individuals develop ways of tapping into the powerful resources of the mind to affect physical, psychological and spiritual change. Patients can gain fulfilment from the part that they feel they have played in controlling events in their lives, although guilt can also be felt if the cancer is not cured. Many patients actively seek to understand and resolve emotional and spiritual pain using relaxation and guided imagery (Kinghorn and Gamlin 2001).

Several researchers suggest that psychological interventions can have a positive effect on survival based on work completed with patients who have skin cancer and haematological malignancies (Walker et al. 1999). Further work with patients with breast cancer suggests that combining relaxation therapy and guided imagery reduces stress and enables patients to respond more positively to the effects of treatment. The treatments actively involve patients in their own care and provide them with some sense of independence, which can promote positive thinking, promote feelings of well-being and help distract patients from dwelling on morbid thoughts (Sloman 2002).

Conclusion

It is clear that complementary therapies can enhance the patient's cancer journey and improve quality of life, in some cases. It does, however, remain important to highlight the care and caution that should be addressed for any therapy. General advice is available on the type of massage used, amount of pressure, caution on cancer-affected areas, and awareness of treatment implications such as skin sensitivity to essential oils and emotional sensitivity related to altered body image.

At the moment, for people with cancer, the above therapies are complementary to orthodox care and should be viewed as enhancing quality of life at every stage of the cancer journey.

References

Farrant A (2003) The time for integration has arrived. Cancer Nurs Pract 2(4): 14–16.

Hann DM, Baker F, Denniston MM (2003) Oncology professionals' communication with cancer patients about complementary therapy: a survey. Complement Ther Med 11: 184–90.

Hodgson H (2000) Does reflexology impact on cancer patients quality of life? Nurs Stand 14(31): 33–8.

Kinghorn S, Gamlin R (eds) (2001) Palliative Nursing: Bringing comfort and hope. London: Baillière Tindall.

Kite SM, Maher EJ, Anderson K et al. (1998) Development of an aromatherapy service at a cancer centre. Palliative Med 12: 171–80.

Macnish S (2001) Complementary therapies. In: Kinghorn S, Gamlin R (eds), Palliative Nursing: Bringing comfort and hope. London: Baillière Tindall.

Peace G, Simons D (1996) Completing the whole. Nurs Times 92(25): 52–4.

Prince of Wales Foundation for Integrated Health and National Council for Hospice and Specialist Palliative Care (2003) National Guidelines for the Use of Complementary Therapies in Supportive and Palliative Care. London: PWFIH and NCHSPC.

Sloman R (2002) Relaxation and guided imagery for anxiety and depression control in community patients with advanced cancer. Cancer Nurs 25: 432–5.

Stevenson C (1996) Complementary therapies in cancer care: an NHS approach. Int J Palliative Nurs 2(1): 15–18.

Walker LG, Walker MB, Oghston K et al. (1999) Psychological, clinical and pathological effects of relaxation training and guided imagery during primary chemotherapy. Br J Cancer 80: 262–8.

Wilcock A, Manderson C, Weller R et al. (2004) Does aromatherapy massage benefit patients with cancer attending a specialist palliative care day centre? Palliative Med 18: 287–90.

Wilkinson S, Aldridge J, Salmon I, Cain E, Wilson B (1999) An evaluation of aromatherapy massage in palliative care. Palliative Med 13: 409–17.

Chapter 10

Pain and symptom management

Pain

Of the many symptoms of cancer, pain is often the most feared, possibly as a result of the fact that unrelieved pain can affect all aspects of a person's life. According to the World Health Organisation (WHO), pain is one of the most common symptoms experienced by people with cancer (WHO 1996). Studies indicate that cancer pain is synonymous with anxiety, fatigue, emotional distress, mood disorders, depression, fewer social interactions and altered family activities (Dorepaal et al. 1989). Relief of pain is essential to improve the quality of life for patients with cancer, yet cancer-related pain is often poorly treated, resulting in unnecessary suffering. Of patients with cancer pain 70–90% could obtain complete relief with oral analgesics, yet moderate-to-severe pain is being reported by 70–80% of them at some stage of the illness (Cleary and Carbone 1995).

Literature suggests that nurses do not possess sufficient knowledge with which to nurse patients in pain and that pain control remains inadequate (Clarke et al. 1996, McCaffery and Ferrell 1997, Drayer et al. 1999). The WHO state that pain can be controlled in 70–90% of cancer patients using relatively inexpensive and simple methods (WHO 1996); however, it has been estimated that adequate control of pain is achieved in only 50% of patients in western societies (Hanks 1994). This chapter aims to give the reader an overview of pain, including an assessment and principles of management. The reader is guided to the numerous books available for in-depth knowledge of physiology and pharmacology.

Acute pain

This has a definite onset, usually as a result of an injury or illness, and its duration is limited and predictable. It is often accompanied by signs of anxiety and by clinical signs of tachycardia, tachypnoea, sweating, dilated pupils and pallor. These signs are considered to be characteristic of individuals in pain (Figure 10.1).

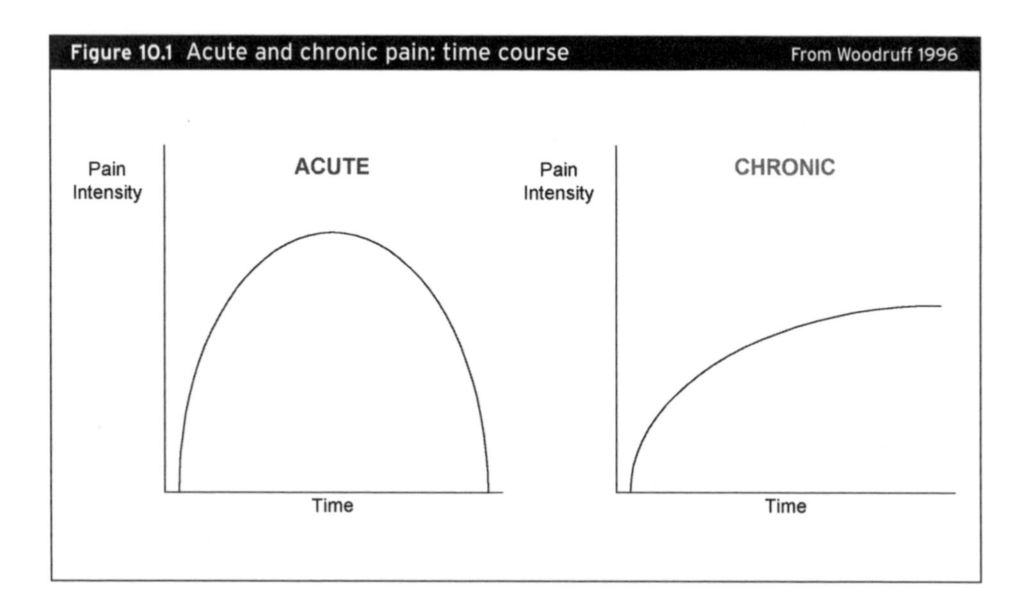

Figure 10.1 Acute and chronic pain: time course From Woodruff 1996

Chronic pain

This differs from acute pain in that it results from a chronic pathological process. The onset is gradual over time and it can become progressively more severe. Individuals often appear depressed or withdrawn and frequently are described as not looking like 'someone in pain'.

Nurses will care for patients experiencing different types of pain. The most common types are covered below.

Types of pain

Neuropathic pain

This pain, also called neurogenic or deafferentation pain, is often hard for patients and staff to understand because there is no obvious noxious stimulus present. This type of pain is the result of current or past damage to the peripheral and/or central nervous system. It can be very unpleasant and long lasting, resulting in loss of sleep, and is described in various ways. Patients often say it is burning, aching or dull in type; however, sharp shooting pains can also be experienced and numbness. Some patients cannot bear clothing to touch the affected area.

Somatic, cutaneous and visceral pain

Somatic pain refers to pain in the musculoskeletal system – namely, bones, periosteum, tendons and fascia.

Visceral pain

This is pain in the internal organs. Internal organs such as the gut are affected by twisting and distension and this causes the pain. Acute visceral pain is often very intense, dull and aching; it is vaguely localized and accompanied by rigid abdominal muscles (guarding), pallor and sweating. Small amounts of visceral pain lead to dramatic autonomic activity (Cervero 1988). The pain that a person experiences is disproportionate to the internal damage. An important point to note is that visceral pain leads to referred pain.

Pain and advanced cancer are not synonymous. Although three-quarters of patients experience pain, a quarter do not (Twycross 1997). Multiple concurrent pains are common in those who have pain:

- A third will have a single pain
- A third will have two pains
- A third will have three or more pains.

Not all cancer pain is caused by the actual cancer (Woodruff 1996):

- 70% is the result of tumour involvement
- 20% is associated with treatment
- < 10% is a result of general illness but not cancer
- < 10% is unrelated to the cancer or its treatment.

Total pain

When discussing pain, it is important to be aware that we should not just be looking at it as a physical dimension. Saunders (1967) introduced the concept of total pain to highlight that pain is multidimensional and that non-physical as well as physical aspects must be addressed: total pain is made up of physical, psychological, social and spiritual aspects.

Pain is also associated with suffering (Figures 10.2–10.4). Unrelieved pain may exacerbate other physical symptoms and vice versa. Problems in other areas can also aggravate pain. These problems need addressing if pain is to be effectively managed and looking at the individual and the family and caring for them in a holistic way can best do this.

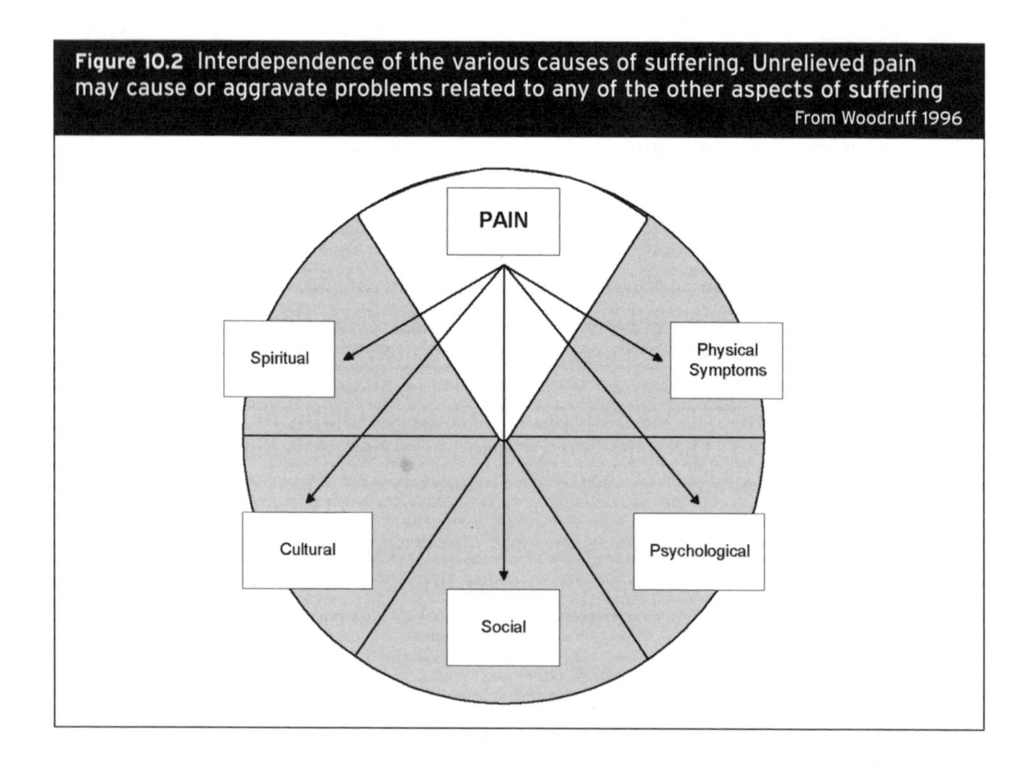

Figure 10.2 Interdependence of the various causes of suffering. Unrelieved pain may cause or aggravate problems related to any of the other aspects of suffering
From Woodruff 1996

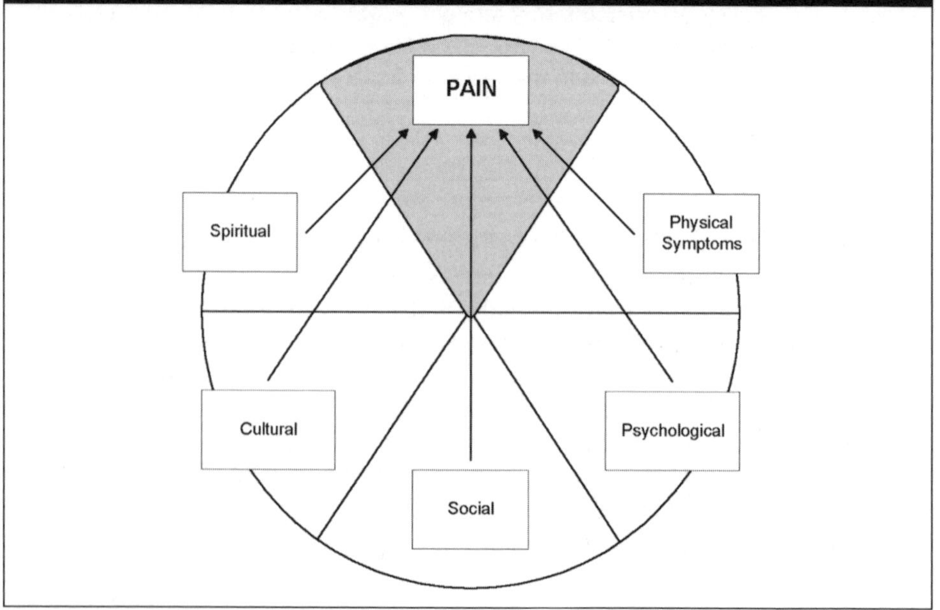

Figure 10.3 Interdependence of the various causes of suffering. Unresolved or untreated problems related to any of the other causes of suffering may cause or aggravate pain
From Woodruff 1996

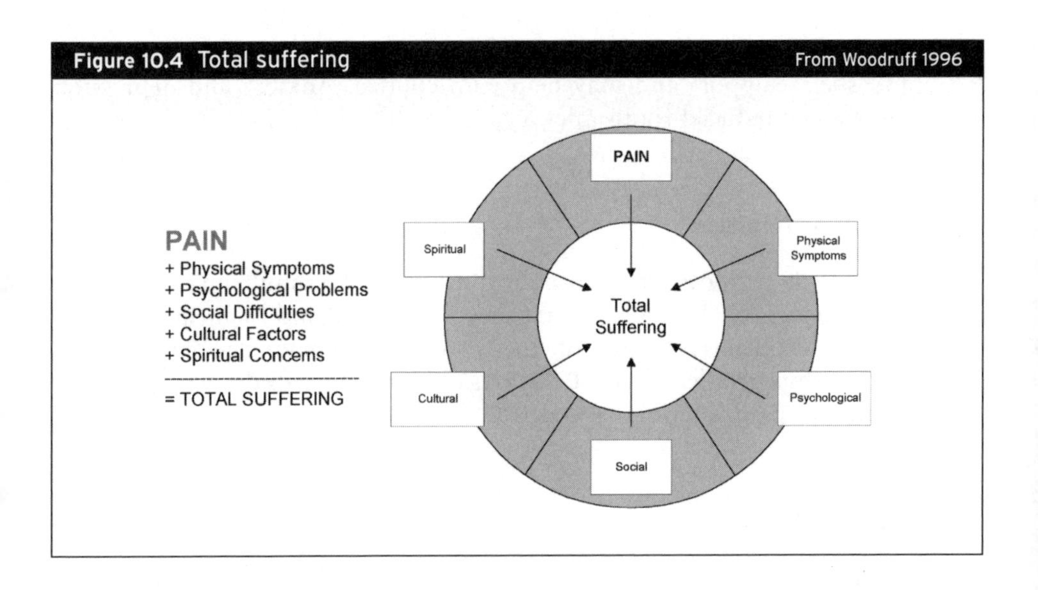

Perception of pain

Pain is:

> ... whatever the experiencing person says it is, existing whenever the experiencing person says it does.
>
> McCaffery and Beebe (1989)

Pain is always subjective. It is important to be aware that other physical symptoms will aggravate the perception of pain so palliation of other symptoms is essential to improve pain control.

Other factors can also affect pain; looking at the individual holistically will ensure that none of these issues is missed.

Psychological problems

These are the most common factors aggravating perception of pain and a failure to recognize and treat psychological distress will worsen an individual's pain. Some clinical features of psychological distress are anxiety, depression and despair. The management of these problems is aimed at helping patients to develop their adaptive and coping mechanisms (Woodruff 1996). This needs to be individualized for each patient.

Counselling could be valuable. Support groups provide both emotional and social support and may help pain control. Anxiety and depression can also be reduced (Bottomley 1997).

Social difficulties

Individuals with cancer are usually a member of a family and have other social networks. This means that they have social and financial responsibilities. Problems in any of these areas, e.g. financial hardship or relationship problems, can lead to isolation and withdrawal, and may mean that pain is harder to control.

Cultural factors

It is important to be aware that different cultures have varying degrees of acceptance of pain, ranging from stoicism to severe anxiety and depression, with some writers suggesting that people in western cultures have lower tolerance of pain (Illich 1976, Menges 1984). Attitudes to pain relief and palliative care also vary. Communication can be made difficult because of language barriers. Culturally sensitive management is essential and can best be achieved by being knowledgeable about the culture and an individual's perception of pain. Interpreters can be used to help with communication.

Spiritual factors

Not to be confused with religion, every individual has his or her own spirituality – this is about meaning and existence. An individual may have regrets or guilt about past events, e.g. about relationships or missed opportunities, and feel that there is no time to rectify these. Allowing patients time to talk or tell their story can help and goes some way to relieving their distress. For those who observe religious practices, there may be specific problems: they may believe that their disease is a punishment. Highfield (1992) highlights that nurses do not assess patients' spiritual needs. Nurses must ensure that this aspect is not overlooked, by discussing it when planning a programme of care, and they should not be afraid of enlisting the help of others, e.g. ministers of religion, in addressing any difficulties. They should, however, recognize that patient and nurses may prefer different spiritual care-givers (Hawthorn and Redmond 1998).

Assessment of pain

Successful management of pain depends on an accurate systemic assessment (de Wit et al. 1999). Recent reviews have, however, found little evidence that this takes place and that assessment is problematic and inconsistent (McCaffery and Ferrell 1997, Rond et al. 1999). Assessment needs to be comprehensive and to include all aspects of pain, not just its severity. Accurate assessment of pain relies on nurses believing the patient's pain rating. Implementation of therapeutic control is not always appropriate to the pain rating, suggesting that nurses may not accept patient reporting of their own pain (McCaffery and Ferrell 1997). Failure to conduct an adequate assessment of pain and documentation of pain management may be interpreted as undertreatment of pain and could result in allegations of serious professional misconduct or litigation (Barrie 2004). Nurses should be aware of their legal responsibilities to ensure accurate documentation (Nursing and Midwifery Council or NMC 2002).

Barriers to adequate assessment

Incorrect interpretation of non-verbal cues can contribute to poor assessment. Nurses may assume that if patients look comfortable or are sleeping they must be pain free because individuals in pain are expected to exhibit certain behaviours and physiological signs. Some pain control behaviours such as watching television, chatting or participating in activities can also be interpreted as signs that the patient is not in pain (Wilkie et al. 1989).

Those who experience more expressible pain behaviours such as crying, moaning or facial expressions of suffering can be perceived by nurses as being more distressed than the stoic patient (Von Baeyer et al. 1984). Assessment of pain is further complicated by nurses assuming that patients will complain of pain, whereas patients expect nurses to enquire about their pain (Seers 1987, Franke and Theeuwen 1994). Poor communication on the part of nurses and patients can hinder assessment, and difficulties can arise when patients are unable to find the words to describe the pain adequately.

Wilkinson (1991) studied nurses communicating with cancer patients and found that they carried out very superficial assessments; thus interventions were planned on the basis of incomplete information. Just as the patient's culture affects the perception of pain, so the nurse's own cultural background may influence the degree to which she or he infers suffering in patients. There is evidence that nurses from various backgrounds differ in their inferences of both physical pain and psychological distress (Davitz and Davitz 1985, McCaffery and Ferrell 1997).

Assessment tools

A comprehensive assessment is essential. There are many different kinds of instruments for assessing the intensity and type of pain and nurses are more knowledgeable than physicians or pharmacists in pain assessment (Furstenburg et al. 1998). The process of assessment should include facilitating the patients to tell their own story through their own perspective (Webb 1992). The simplest measures of pain and those most widely used are the visual analogue scale (VAS) and the verbal pain rating scale. The VAS (Figure 10.5) is an easy and simple tool for the assessment of pain and the measurement of pain intensity. It is important that the same kind of instrument is always used with the same patient. Daily pain ratings are essential to ensure continuity and it is important that the information is documented. Evidence shows that recordings of ratings are often inconsistent (Graffam 1990).

Pictorial records (Figure 10.6) of the site of pain can be completed by either patients or nurses; however, it should be noted that patients and nurses differ in their assessment of the most intense level of pain suffered by

Figure 10.5 Self-report measures for pain severity — From Woodruff 1996

Visual Analogue Scale

Instruction: mark on the line below how strong your pain is

no pain -- worst possible pain

Numerical Rating Scale

Instruction: on a scale of 1 to 10, how strong is your pain?

no pain = 0 - 1 - 2 - 3 - 4 - 5 - 6 - 7 - 8 - 9 - 10 = worst pain possible

Verbal Descriptor Scale

Instruction: which word best describes your pain?

None Mild Moderate Severe Excruciating

patients, with nurses believing that their patients accept and tolerate more pain than the patients themselves say is the case (Hovi and Lauri 1999).

Figure 10.6 Pictorial record: the patient is asked to indicate the site of the pain or it may be completed by the examining doctor or nurse From Woodruff 1996

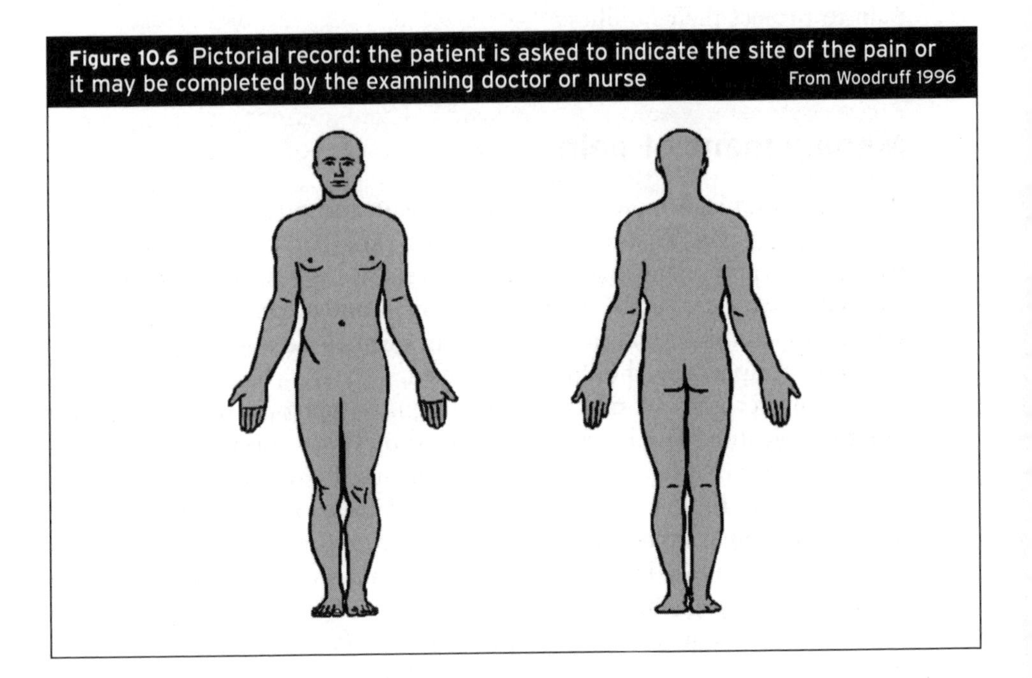

Despite the benefits of assessing pain, many nurses resist using the tools. Common criticisms are that using the tools takes too long and some nurses feel that their own judgement is satisfactory. However, nursing a patient with unmanaged pain takes far longer, so time taken to assess is worthwhile. Relying on one's own judgement can be dangerous if the practitioner is a novice in this field because information may be missed; using a tool can help ensure that nothing is missed (Gordon 1987). It is also important to use a tool to ensure consistency because the same nurse is not on duty 24 hours a day, 7 days a week. Others argue that assessment tools in use are not relevant to their clinical area, in which case the tools can be adapted to suit the situation.

Just carrying out an assessment is pointless unless the information obtained is used in clinical decision-making. So a finding that a patient has high blood pressure or temperature will trigger the nurse to take action, as should a high pain assessment scoring. Tools are also very helpful in evaluating the effectiveness of the pain management programme. As a result of the subjective nature of pain, it is extremely likely that the carer's and the health-care professional's perceptions will differ from the patient's direct experience of pain. It may be that family members may be reluctant to acknowledge pain for fear that the disease is progressing (Barrie 2004). Houts et al. (1996) found that patients often under-reported pain to protect their families.

Management of pain

Good communication with both the patient and other members of the caring team will ensure a coordinated approach to pain control. Reassuring the patient that pain can be relieved is essential. Patients are entitled to expect effective pain management and a total absence of pain wherever possible. As all aspects of pain need to be addressed, a multidisciplinary approach should be employed.

As pain becomes worse, when it occupies a person's whole attention other interventions can be used. Evidence shows that non-pharmacological interventions are effective in the management of pain and nurses should consider using these in pain management (Sindhu 1996, Wallace 1997); despite this, nurses tend not to use these approaches (Ferrell et al. 1991, Franke et al. 1996). Diversional activities can be used because they do more than just pass the time; nurses can encourage patients to watch television, read or converse. If pain persists, modification to a patient's way of life and environment may be required. The help of the physiotherapist and occupational therapist is often valuable.

The multifaceted nature of pain means that it is unlikely that pharmacological interventions will relieve it entirely. Nurses can use other pain control interventions such as distraction, massage or the application of heat quite easily in their everyday practice to benefit patients. Poor positioning can also exacerbate pain; helping patients who are bed-bound to maintain a comfortable position with the use of pillows and other supports, and minimizing the number of times that they have to move, are important interventions (Hawthorn and Redmond 1998). Evidence shows, however, that nurses tend not to do so (Ferrell et al. 1991, Fothergill-Bourbonnais and Wilson Barnett 1992, Franke et al. 1996). The following focuses briefly on such interventions.

Massage

Massage has been used as a therapeutic intervention for thousands of years. It can have a direct physiological effect on pain, reducing muscle spasm and tension. Carers can be taught simple massage techniques, which can help overcome feelings of helplessness. Before attempting to use massage, it must first be ascertained whether touch is acceptable to the patient because it may cause anxiety and discomfort in those who dislike physical touch (Hawthorn and Redmond 1998). Concern has been expressed that massage may encourage the spread of cancer (McNamara 1994); however, although there is no evidence to support this belief, it is not wise to massage directly over a palpable tumour or an area undergoing radiotherapy.

Reflexology

Reflexology is a treatment that has a basis in massage. It can be performed on the feet or hands and used to treat various disorders. Applying gently pressure to these areas may reduce pain and anxiety. Basic foot massage can be taught to carers and this will allow them to be involved in care (Whitlock 1999)

Heat treatment

Heat treatment can be used effectively to relieve pain, offering a simple and cost-effective non-pharmacological intervention for pain (Hawthorn and Redmond 1998). The superficial application of heat increases the blood flow to the skin and superficial organs, which will improve tissue oxygenation and nutrition, and aid in the elimination of pain-causing substances (Hawthorn and Redmond 1998). It is of particular benefit in the treatment of muscle spasms and the musculoskeletal discomforts that are associated with immobility and debility. As heat treatment can cause tissue damage, care should be taken where there is diminished sensation or paralysis; it should also be avoided in the presence of infection. Heat treatment can be achieved with hot packs, hot water bottles, electric heating pads, radiant heat lamps and hydrotherapy.

Although there is controversy surrounding the use of superficial heat in cancer patients, with some expressing concern that it facilitates tumour growth and metastatic spread, evidence to support this view is limited and the use of superficial heat to control pain can still be recommended (Jacox et al. 1994)

Cold therapy

Cold therapy, the superficial application of cold, causes vasoconstriction of the skin and blood vessels, and helps prevent or reduce swelling after injury. It can also decrease the production of pain-causing metabolites and conduction in pain fibres (Ernst and Fialka 1994). Cold is thought to be more effective, has a shorter duration of application, works quicker and produces a longer-lasting effect than heat (Hawthorn and Redmond 1998). Unfortunately many people are averse to cold and find heat much more acceptable (McCaffery 1990). Cold therapy can be applied in the form of icepacks, ethyl chloride spray or immersion in iced water.

The application of both heat and cold is contraindicated in areas that have previously been treated with radiotherapy (Hawthorn and Redmond 1998).

Music therapy

According to Larsen-Beck (1991) music can ameliorate pain by means of distraction, reduction of anxiety, counter-stimulation and increased feelings of control. It has also been shown to be effective at reducing pain in oncology (Zimmerman et al. 1989, Larsen-Beck 1991). Nurses can help by offering patients a range of different music to listen to, with headphones to block out distracting noise.

Environment

An unpleasant environment and loss of privacy have been cited as factors contributing to pain (Faggerhaugh and Strauss 1977, Wainwright 1985). Allowing patients control over lighting, temperature and ventilation can help, as can affording them privacy. It may be difficult for patients to express their pain in a busy ward and this makes assessment difficult. A pleasant environment facilitates rest and thus can help in the alleviation of pain (Fordham and Dunn 1994). Achieving this in a hospital is difficult; however, that should not deter health professionals from trying.

Education of patients and families

The nurse has a pivotal role to play in the education of patients and families. Myths and misconceptions about pain and treatment abound and this can result in patients either refusing to take analgesics or increasing the dose. Patients who receive drug-related education have improved pain relief, better compliance with pain medication regimens and less concern about taking opioids than patients who have not received such education (Rimer et al. 1992). Families also have a need for information, especially if they are involved in the care of the patient at home. Family members often have to decide what pain medication to give, how much to give and when to give it (Ferrell et al. 1991). It is important to remember that their response to expressions of pain can ameliorate or exacerbate it (Ferrell et al. 1991); thus patient and family education is an on-going process, not a one-off event.

Nurses need to give patients taking a number of different medications the following information:

- Written instructions to take home with them.
- Warning about possible side effects, because experiencing these when medication is first started may lead to a discontinuation.
- Contact telephone numbers should be given to patients and they should be advised to call if they have any concerns.

Analgesic programmes should be kept as simple as possible and any fears about dependence and addiction need to be discussed. Patients are often anxious when prescribed morphine thinking that they will soon die or that nothing will be left when the pain gets worse. They need reassurance that morphine can be used for months or years and is compatible with a normal lifestyle, and also that the therapeutic range is such that the dosage can be increased if necessary.

Principles of pain relief

These principles are covered in this section, and again the reader is guided to books on pharmacology for more detailed guidance, e.g. Twycross (1994).

Satisfactory pain relief can be achieved in 95% of patients with cancer. It is best to aim for:

- pain relief at night
- pain relief at rest during the day
- pain relief on movement (recognizing that this is not always possible).

The oral route is the preferred route and analgesics should be given regularly and prophylactically, never 'as required'. The World Health Organization's three-step analgesic ladder should be used (Figure 10.7).

Examples of drugs to be used at each stage are (Woodruff 1996):

- Step 1: aspirin or non-steroidal anti-inflammatories
- Step 2: codeine or oxycodeine
- Step 3: morphine or methadone.

Figure 10.7 World Health Organization's three-step ladder (WHO 1996)

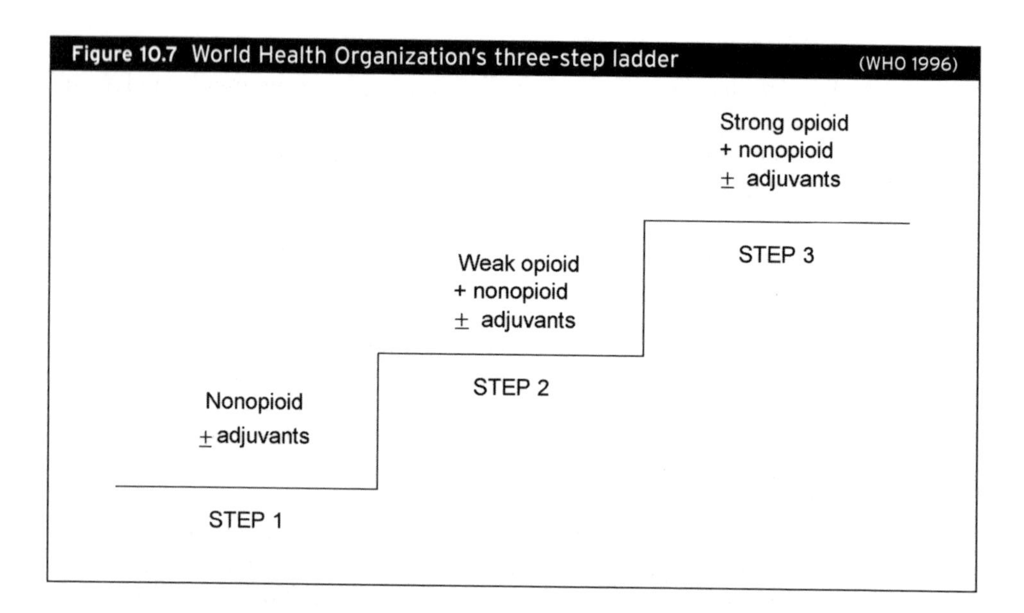

Adjuvant drugs

Adjuvant drugs Hawthorn and Redmond (1998) should be used, e.g. laxatives are always required with morphine usage. An adjuvant drug is, strictly speaking, one that potentiates the action of another, e.g. adjuvant anxiolytic may be given alongside an analgesic to reduce anxiety and this will also help pain relief.

Antidepressant drugs

Antidepressant drugs have also been shown to be analgesic for a wide variety of painful conditions, e.g. headache or chronic facial pain, and can be useful in patients with high levels of anxiety.

Steroids

Steroids reduce oedema and thus can be useful in relieving visceral pain and bone pain, because they relieve pressure on compressed structures. The analgesic effect is accompanied by an increase in appetite and well-being.

Anticonvulsants

Anticonvulsants can be useful in the treatment of neuropathic pain, although the mechanism of action is unknown.

Although detailed description of all medication used to relieve pain is beyond the scope of this section, it is important that nurses have a good knowledge of pain medication. Hovi and Lauri (1999) found that nurses with poor knowledge of morphine and its use in pain management tended to underestimate the patient's most intense experiences of pain.

Points to be aware of are that morphine usage is dictated by therapeutic need, not by prognosis and, in cancer patients, it does not cause clinically important respiratory depression. The use of morphine does not, however, guarantee success in pain relief if the psychosocial aspects of care are ignored.

Fatigue

Fatigue is one of the most commonly reported symptoms of cancer and its treatment, particularly related to radiotherapy, chemotherapy and advancing disease (Kuzbit 2002, Porock and Palmer 2004). Fatigue in cancer care is often mismanaged or not managed at all, mainly because of staff and patient perceptions of fatigue as an inevitable symptom of the disease and its treatment. Cancer-related fatigue, as opposed to general fatigue, tends to have a rapid onset with a greater intensity and is of longer duration.

Fatigue is often described by patients as an overwhelming whole body and mind tiredness, unrelieved by sleep or rest, and changing in its nature with disease progression or advancing treatments. According to experts in this area, fatigue is multidimensional and subjective, affecting the patient's physical well-being and impacting on psychological, social and spiritual health (Ferrell et al. 1996, Richardson and Ream 1996, Kuzbit 2002). Reported effects of fatigue include:

- tiredness
- lack of energy
- general lethargy
- weakness
- exhaustion
- inability to sustain exertion
- impaired mobility
- reduced motivation
- reduced attention span
- sleepiness
- drowsiness
- heaviness
- apathy
- an inability to continue.

Management of cancer-related fatigue is based around the concept that fatigue arises as a result of inactivity and decreased functioning. Methods to address this are aimed at alleviating primary symptoms and managing secondary fatigue, with a balance of rest and activity. Assessment is key to the management of cancer-related fatigue as it is for the management of other symptoms. The problem with assessing fatigue is its lack of recognition as a symptom by patients and health-care professionals alike. Several assessment tools are available but are infrequently used. Where assessment is used it is often as part of a general assessment checklist and, as has been stated, fatigue is not always recognized as a major symptom. In reality fatigue, if mismanaged, has a huge impact on the quality of life of the cancer patient.

Interventions in the management of fatigue concentrate on four main areas:

1. Exercise: general gentle exercise offers useful aerobic activity and is linked to a sense of well-being.
2. Activity: this does not necessarily just mean the general, mundane, day-to-day activity involved in activities of daily living, but includes hobbies and pastimes that are perceived as being enjoyable.
3. Education: education about cancer-related fatigue is important in order for patients to understand why they are feeling tired and the fact that tiredness is not always related to disease progression.
4. Psychosocial intervention: this may include music therapy, relaxation and guided imagery.

Fatigue in cancer care is a debilitating problem. Care should be focused on holistic individualized assessment and management, in order to improve health-care professionals' understanding of fatigue and enhance quality of life for the patient.

Gastrointestinal symptom management

Anorexia

Illness, hospitalization and surgery all increase the body's nutritional demands, as does cancer and its treatment. The last can also cause problems with supplying nutritional demand. Appetite can be affected in several ways as a result of altered glucose metabolism, changes in the muscle of the stomach wall and treatments such as morphine. Effects include:

- Altered sense of taste and smell
- Early satiety or sense of fullness

- Delayed gastric emptying
- Nausea and vomiting
- Conditioned food aversions (related to certain drugs or treatments)
- Physical problems with eating related to the mouth, oesophagus or other parts of the gastrointestinal system
- Anxiety
- Depression
- Pain
- Stress.

Management of anorexia should be implemented along the cancer pathway. At the start of treatment, for those with little or no weight loss, information about loss of appetite and balanced diets as well as diet supplements can be given. For patients who are unable to eat as a result of an inability to swallow, enteral feeding is recommended. For those patients in whom the gastrointestinal tract is not functioning at all, as a result of the disease process, parenteral nutrition may be more appropriate. In palliative care it may be advantageous to increase the appetite with a stimulant, although in some cases a higher than usual calorie intake may increase tumour metabolism.

In all situations patients should be encouraged to:

- eat something that they like
- eat small meals more often
- eat high-protein foods
- allow others to cook
- stimulate appetite with exercise when able
- use food diaries
- take appropriate medication for the relief of pain, nausea and constipation
- look after the mouth.

Health-care professionals need an understanding of the physiology of nutrition as well as the social significance of food in order to provide optimal care. Nutritional assessment is key to providing optimal care. Eating is linked to spiritual experiences, social activity and symbolism. In the context of illness, eating, refusal to eat or weight loss will have great significance (Walsh 1999, Corner and Bailey 2001).

Nausea and vomiting

Nausea and vomiting are two of the most common and most distressing side effects of cancer and its treatment. In some cases the symptoms are so severe that patients feel unable or unwilling to carry on with treatment.

A wide variety of physiological and psychological causes may result in nausea and vomiting:

- Mechanical obstruction of the gut
- Increased pressure in the brain as a result of tumour load, oedema or electrolyte imbalance
- Radiotherapy
- Chemotherapy
- Antibiotics
- Conditioned response to smells, foods, treatments (anticipatory nausea and vomiting).

The management of this distressing symptom should begin with some understanding of the enormity of the problem to the individual. Clear and careful assessment of the problem should then follow, with subsequent management and evaluation. Management of nausea and vomiting can include pharmacological and non-pharmacological strategies. Non-pharmacological strategies may include patient education and information, music therapy, humour, exercise, hypnosis, guided imagery and relaxation. A wide variety of pharmacological agents is now used to prevent and treat nausea and vomiting. Single and combination drugs are used, the drug of choice, dose, frequency and route of administration being adjusted according to the severity of the nausea and vomiting experienced.

Constipation and diarrhoea

Altered bowel habit can be a symptom of cancer and its treatment and, if not managed effectively, can lead to bowel obstruction, dehydration, electrolyte imbalance, nausea, anorexia, pain, general malaise and social isolation. Causes of constipation are:

- Decreased fibre intake
- Decreased fluid intake
- Lack of exercise/mobility
- Tumour load
- Drug therapy
- Surgery
- Lack of privacy
- Interruption of normal bowel pattern.

Causes of diarrhoea are:

- Chemotherapy
- Radiotherapy

- Surgery
- Nutritional supplements
- Antibiotics
- Anxiety.

Management of this symptom should again include clear assessment. A cancer history should be taken as well as elimination patterns, medication, diet history, exercise activity and medication. Pharmacological interventions to rectify the constipation or diarrhoea should be used together with identification of the main causative factors. If, for example, chemotherapy is the main causative factor, that treatment may need to be altered or reduced until symptoms are under control. Fluid intake, at least 2 l/day, and foods high in fibre should be encouraged in patients who have constipation or diarrhoea. Management of skin problems, particularly related to diarrhoea, should be addressed as well as sensitive social management (Nevidjon and Sowers 2001).

Mucositis

Mucositis is the inflammation, ulceration and ultimately the destruction of mucosal cells. Mucosal cells line the gastrointestinal, genitourinary and respiratory tracts. In the management of cancer the effects of mucositis in the gastrointestinal tract are most common, particularly in the area of the oral cavity.

Mucositis can affect a patient's quality of life and ability to continue with treatment and, as with the management of other symptoms, has an impact on the cost of care (Nevidjon and Sowers 2001).

The main causes of mucositis are the effects of chemotherapy and radiotherapy; as well as destroying cancer cells, the rapidly dividing cells of the mucosa are also damaged. Poor nutrition, dehydration and poor oral hygiene are contributory factors, as well as interventions such as oxygen therapy and other drugs that dry the mucous membranes.

Again assessment is the key to good management and should include questions related to the following as well as visualization of the mouth:

- Pain
- Changes in taste
- Changes in saliva
- Sensation
- Ability to swallow
- Ability to speak
- Discoloured areas
- Treatment history.

Management will include antibiotic therapy, if necessary, analgesia, increased fluid intake, and good oral care, including care of teeth or dentures, the oral cavity itself and the lips.

Conclusion

There is evidence to suggest that the quality of the cancer experience affects not only the patient but also those close to him or her. A consistent concern of families is the need for the patient to receive pain relief and adequate comfort and care. Families, who witness the suffering or uncontrolled pain of a relative, experience suffering themselves. For patients and their families, quality of life will be maximized in situations where the goals of pain and symptom management are valued. Services should be responsive to patients' needs with the central role of families acknowledged as well as the importance of primary and community services. Good communication between health-care professionals within the multidisciplinary team will result in expert pain and symptom management and enhanced quality of life for all (Ferrell et al. 1991, Kristjanson and Avery 1994, National Institute for Clinical Effectiveness or NICE 2004).

References

Barrie J (2004) The value of thorough assessment in the management of cancer pain. Prof Nurse 19: 446–8.

Bottomley A (1997) Cancer support groups: are they effective? Eur J Cancer 6: 11–17.

Cervero F (1988) Visceral pain. In: Dubvier R, Gebhart FG, Bond MR (eds), Proceedings of the Fifth World Conference on Pain. Amsterdam: Elsevier Science Publishers, pp. 216–26.

Clarke E, French B, Bilodeau M, Capasso V, Edwards A, Empolili J (1996) Pain management knowledge, attitudes and clinical practice: the impact of nurses' characteristics and education. J Pain Symptom Manag 11: 18–31.

Cleary J, Carbone PP (1995) Pharmacologic management of cancer pain. Hosp Practit 30(11): 41–9.

Corner J, Bailey C (eds) (2001) Cancer Nursing Care in Context. Oxford: Blackwell

Davitz LL, Davitz JR (1985) Culture and nurses' inferences of suffering. In: Copp LA (ed.), Recent Advances in Nursing: Perspectives on pain. Edinburgh: Churchill Livingstone, pp. 17–28.

de Wit R, Van Dam F, Vielvoye-Kerkmeer A, Mattern C, Abu-Saad HH (1999) The treatment of chronic pain in a cancer hospital in the Netherlands. J Pain Symptom Manag 17: 333–50.

Dorepaal KL, Aaronson NK, Van dam FSAM (1989) Pain experience and pain management among hospitalised cancer patients. A clinical study. Cancer 63: 593–8.

Drayer RA, Henderson BS, Reidenberg M (1999) Barriers to better pain controlling hospitalised patients. J Pain Symptom Manag 17: 434–40.

Ernst E, Fialka V (1994) Ice freezes pain? A review of the clinical effectiveness of analgesic cold therapy. J Pain Symptom Manag 9: 56–9.
Faggerhaugh SY, Strauss A (1977) Politics of Pain Management. Staff-patient interaction. Los Angeles, CA: Addison-Wesley.
Ferrell BA, Zichi Cohen M, Rhiner M, Rozek A (1991) Pain as a metaphor for illness. Part II Family care givers management of pain. Oncol Nurs Forum 18: 1315–21.
Ferrell BR, Grant M, Dean GE, Funk B, Ly J (1996) 'Bone tired': the experience of fatigue and its impact on quality of life. Oncol Nurs Forum 23: 1539–47.
Fordham M, Dunn S (1994) Alongside the Person in Pain. London: Baillière Tindall.
Fothergill-Bourbonnais F, Wilson Barnett J (1992) A comparative study of intensive therapy unit and hospice nurses' knowledge of pain management. J Adv Nurs 17: 362–72.
Franke AL, Theeuwen I (1994) Inhibition in expressing pain: a qualitative study among Dutch surgical breast cancer patients. Cancer Nurs 17: 193–9.
Franke AL, Garssen B, Abu Saad H, Grypdonck M (1996) Qualitative needs assessment prior to a continuing education program. J Cont Educ Nurs 27: 34–41.
Furstenburg C, Ahles TA, Whedon MB et al. (1998) Knowledge and attitudes of health care providers toward cancer pain management. A comparison of physicians, nurses and pharmacists in the state of New Hampshire. J Pain Symptom Manag 15: 335–49.
Gordon M (1987) Nursing Diagnosis: Process and application. New York: McGraw-Hill.
Graffam S (1990) Pain content in the curriculum. A survey. Nurse Educator 15(1): 20–3.
Hanks GW (1994) Palliative medicine problem areas in pain and symptom management. Cancer Surv 21: 1–3.
Hawthorn J, Redmond K (1998) Pain: Causes and management. London: Blackwell Science.
Highfield MF (1992) Spiritual health of oncology patients: nurse and patients' perspectives. Cancer Nurs 15: 1–8.
Houts P, Nezu A, Nezu C, Bucher J (1996) The prepared family care giver: a problem solving approach to family caregiver education. Patient Educ Counsel 27: 63–73.
Hovi SL, Lauri S (1999) Patients and nurser assessment of cancer pain. Eur J Cancer Care 8: 213–19.
Illich I (1976) Limits to Medicine: Medical nemesis. The expropriation of health. London: Marion Boyars.
Jacox A, Carr DB, Payne R et al. (1994) Management of Cancer Pain, Clinical Practice Guideline No. 9, Agency for Health Care Policy and Research. Rockville, MD: AHCPR.
Kristjanson LJ Avery L (1994) Vicarious pain: the family's perspective. Pain Manage Newsletter 7(3): 1–2.
Kuzbit P (2002) Improving the patient's experience of cancer related fatigue. Cancer Nurs Pract 1(9): 31–6.
Larsen-Beck S (1991) The therapeutic use of music for cancer-related pain. Oncol Nurs Forum 18: 1327–37.
McCaffery M (1990) Nursing approaches to non-pharmacological pain control. Int J Nurs Studies 27(1): 1–5.
McCaffery M, Beebe A (1989) Pain: A clinical manual for nursing practice. St Louis, MO: CV Mosby Co.
McCaffery M, Ferrell B (1997) Nurses' knowledge of pain assessment and management: how much progress have we made? J Pain Symptom Manage 14: 175–88.
McNamara P (1994) Massage for People with Cancer. London: Wandsworth Cancer Support Centre.
Menges LJ (1984) Pain: still an intriguing puzzle. Soc Sci Med 19: 1257–60.
National Institute for Clinical Effectiveness (2004) Improving Supportive and Palliative Care for Adults with Cancer. London: NICE.
Nevidjon BM, Sowers KW (2001) A Nurse's Guide to Cancer Care. Philadelphia, PA: Lippincott.
Nursing and Midwifery Council (2002) Guidelines for Record Keeping. London: NMC.
Porock D, Palmer D (2004) Cancer of the Gastrointestinal Tract. London: Whurr.

Richardson A, Ream E (1996) The experience of fatigue and other symptoms in patients receiving chemotherapy. Eur J Cancer Care 5(suppl 2): 24–30.
Rimer BK, Kedziera P, Levy MH (1992) The role of patient education in cancer pain. Hospice J 8: 171–91.
Rond ME, de Wit R, de Dam et al. (1999) Daily pain assessment: value for nurses and patients. J Adv Nurs 29: 436–44.
Saunders C (1967) The Management of Terminal Illness. London: Hospice Medicine Publications.
Seers K (1987) Perceptions of pain. Nurs Times 83: 37–9.
Sindhu F (1996) Are non-pharmacological nursing interventions for the management of pain effective? A meta-analysis. J Adv Nurs 24: 1152–9.
Twycross R (1994) Pain Relief in Advanced Cancer. Edinburgh: Churchill Livingstone.
Twycross R (1997) Symptom Management in Advanced Cancer, 2nd edn. Oxford: Radcliffe Medical Press.
Von Baeyer CL, Johnson MG, McMillan MJ (1984) Consequences of non-verbal expression of pain: patient distress and observer concern. Soc Sci Med 19: 1319–24
Wainwright P (1985) Impact of hospital architecture on the patient in pain. In: Acop L (ed.), Recent Advances in Nursing Perspectives on Pain. Edinburgh: Churchill Livingstone, pp. 46–61.
Wallace KG (1997) Analysis of recent literature concerning relaxation and imagery interventions for cancer pain. Cancer Nurs 17: 200–6.
Walsh M (ed.) (1999) Watson's Clinical Nursing and Related Sciences, 5th edn. London: Baillière Tindall.
Webb P (1992) Teaching patients and relatives. In: Tiffany R, Webb P (eds), Oncology for Nurses and Health Care Professionals, 2nd edn. Beaconsfield: Chapman & Hall, pp. 86–101.
Whitlock K (1999) Complementary therapies. In: Aranda S, O'Connor M (eds), Palliative Care Nursing. A guide to practice. Melbourne: Ausmed Publications. pp. 259–73.
Wilkie DJ, Lovejoy N, Dodd MJ, Tesler MD (1989) Pain control behaviours of patients with cancer. In: Funk SG, Tornquist EM, Champagne MT, Copp LA, Wise RA (eds), Management of Pain, Fatigue and Nausea. New York: Springer Publishing Co.
Wilkinson S (1991) Factors which influence how nurses communicate with cancer patients. J Adv Nurs 16: 677–88.
Woodruff R (1996) Cancer Pain. Melbourne: Asperula Pty Ltd.
World Health Organization (1996) Cancer Pain Relief. Geneva: WHO.
Zimmerman L, Pozehl B, Duncan K et al. (1989) Effects of music in patients' who had chronic cancer pain. West J Nurs Res 11: 298–309.

Chapter 11

Body image and sexuality

Body image is a subjective phenomenon, not just based on the individual's perceived physical appearance, but shaped by emotions, social interactions with others and cultural norms. Individuals assess their body image in terms of self-satisfaction but also in relation to others who influence them and act as a social mirror (Corner and Bailey 2001). An altered physical body image affects the individual not just in the physical sense but also in an emotive and social context when influenced by the reactions of others.

Sexuality encompasses the body image we have of ourselves, our self-esteem and how we wish others to see us. It involves sexual desire, activity and orientation, as well as touch, intimacy and the physical closeness of others.

Body image

According to Price (1990) body image refers to three essential components:

1. Body reality: the way in which we perceive and how we feel about our bodies – the body as seen and measured as objectively as possible. Some changes to body reality occur as part of normal development, e.g. during puberty.
2. Body presentation: how the body responds to how we want it to be. This includes the dressing and adornment of the body as well as posture and movement.
3. Body ideal: how we judge the body reality and body presentation; body reality is constantly measured against an ideal that we hold in our heads. Body ideal includes personal space, body size and weight, body strength and function, and body contours. Modern western societies have developed norms of body ideal based on the premise that to be happy one must look and feel young. This message is underpinned by the fashion and advertising industries that increasingly use younger people to promote their products.

Body image changes throughout life, sometimes in relation to illness or disfigurement; when one body image component changes the others will attempt to accommodate the changes that have taken place (Price 1990).

Body image is also affected by self-image, our own assessment of our social worth, composed of ideas of whether we are true to ourselves, and what we perceive that others think of us.

A cancer diagnosis will affect body image and self-image in several ways; cancer development may cause changes to bodily functions and altered body sensations. Pain and symptoms can act as a constant reminder of illness and can cause intense anxiety and emotional suffering. Feelings about the body can blur into anguish about the very nature of existence (Corner and Bailey 2001). The feeling that the body is out of control, something to fear and dislike, may grow with a cancer diagnosis until identity, status, competence and power are all called into question.

People are affected in different ways according to how much of their identity is invested in different parts of their bodies and how cancer and its treatment impact onto this. A young woman might find hair loss intolerable whereas a young man might not mind so much, although this of course is very individual and also culturally dependent. Any form of disfiguring disease or mutilating surgery can lead to body image problems if the person is unable to tolerate or adjust to a changed appearance. A period of mourning can occur for the changed body, often involving self-doubt, a loss of self-esteem and, for some, feelings of depression. Changes in a person's appearance require other people to adjust; relationships sometimes need to be renegotiated, which can sometimes lead to relationship problems and sexual difficulties (Brennan 2004).

Management of body image

As in other areas of cancer care, one of the key ways to support patients is to communicate, to offer clear information, to make oneself available by giving time and being non-judgemental. A useful acronym to encourage patients to use is HAPPINESS (Nevidjon and Sowers 2000):

- **H** for hope: hold on to hope, there is always hope for a pain free day or precious time with a loved one.
- **A** for ask: always ask for help.
- **P** for plan: plan time to do what you want to do.
- **P** for permission: permit experimentation, e.g. with clothes or sexually.
- **I** for image: use touch, massage and affirmation to find the new you.
- **N** for needs: put your own needs before those of others.
- **E** for express: express yourself fully; if it is too difficult to talk about, use a journal.

- **S** for support: find a support group.
- **S** for self: you need to love yourself before others can love you.

Management of body image is a process that evolves through contact with the patient and will involve the multidisciplinary team. Care aimed at supporting the patient with body image issues cannot always be separated from care aimed at other problems. For some patients, body image problems may be the greatest problem of all and support in this area, even if there is no resolution, can have the most profound and long-lasting effect on the patient's life and on the cancer journey (Price 1990).

Sexuality

Sexuality is a person's sense of him- or herself as a desired or desiring object and is directly related to a sense of well-being. Sexuality is influenced by personality, role, relationships, society and culture. Sexuality is integral to quality of life and the issue of sexuality and the cancer patient is well recognized. There is a wealth of literature on sexuality in general, as well as in cancer care, much of which is around its avoidance by health-care professionals who still find issues of a sexual nature difficult to discuss (Van Der Riet 1998, Nevidjon and Sowers 2000, Corner and Bailey 2001).

Sexuality and sexual functioning can be affected physically, psychologically and emotionally at any stage of the cancer journey even before diagnosis. Changes in body functioning and appearance, e.g. as in weight loss or pain, can have an impact on body image, self-esteem, self-confidence and sexual expression. In some patients loss or mutilation of a sexual organ can severely affect body image, manhood or womanhood; for others the threat of death from cancer offers a different perspective and the loss is welcomed. Relationships and sexual functioning can be disrupted; a partner's affection and acceptance can have a big impact on how well the patient adjusts (Mick et al. 2004).

Sexuality can be impinged upon at every point of the disease trajectory. One can feel sexually unattractive as a result of:

- hair loss
- nausea and vomiting
- fatigue
- surgery
- hormonal symptoms such as vaginal dryness and hot flushes
- radiotherapy which can cause skin fibrosis and loss of sensation (women with radiotherapy to the breast)

- experience (by men) of ejaculatory and erectile difficulty as a result of surgery and radiotherapy (Corner and Bailey 2001).

The management of sexuality in cancer patients is difficult and not just based around the cancer diagnosis. The patient's premorbid sexual functioning and relationships will impact on psychosexual adjustment after diagnosis and treatment. The impact of a cancer diagnosis can highlight previous sexual or relationship difficulties. To support patients in this area a knowledgeable and non-judgemental approach is necessary. Health-care professionals need to be comfortable and confident with attitudes and behaviours that are possibly different from their own, with skilled communication being central to the care offered.

Management of sexuality

There are several strategies and models available to support health-care professionals in caring for patients' sexual needs.

The PLISSIT model provides a framework for health-care professionals to work through with their patients, offering different interventions at different stages:

- **P** for permission: allowing patients to feel at ease with their own sexuality. A useful starting point to broach the subject can be at assessment; cues must be taken from the patient, who may not wish to discuss sexuality at that point, but giving permission to do so will not be forgotten.
- **LI** for limited information: this refers to keeping information to a minimum and relevant to the immediate situation that is of concern to the patient.
- **SS** for specific suggestions: refers to information for possible strategies to help overcome the immediate problems related to the disease and its treatment. Specific advice may include management of particular symptoms but may also include information on alternative sexual positions or modification of sexual activity.
- **IT** for intensive therapy: this relates to specialist intervention. Health-care professionals must recognize their own limitations and know which services are available for referral.

Clinical supervision is crucial so that health-care professionals feel supported and gain in confidence and competence in this area (Corner and Bailey 2001).

The BETTER model is similar to PLISSIT and provides information that allows health-care professionals to provide information and conduct sexuality assessments (Mick et al. 2004):

- **B**: bring up the topic.
- **E**: explain that you are concerned with sexuality issues and that patients may talk to you about any concerns that they may have, although you personally might not be able to answer all of their questions.
- **T**: tell patients that you will refer them to someone more suitable if you cannot address their concerns.
- **T** for timing: make it clear that the patient can ask sexuality-related questions at any time.
- **E**: educate patients about the anticipated side effects of their treatment.
- **R**: record assessment and any interventions.

According to Shell (1995), support of patients so that they can maintain an intimate relationship during their cancer journey may allow them and their partners moments of freedom from thoughts of the cancer. Although sexuality might be the 'uninvited guest' in the nurse–patient relationship, neither stops being a sexual being when immersed in those roles. In caring for our patients we also need to care for ourselves and be aware of our own sexuality before we can be aware of the sexuality of others (Quinn 2003).

Conclusion

A changed experience of the body, when it is damaged, mutilated, incomplete or spoilt in some way, can deeply affect one's sense of self with accompanying feelings of isolation, fragmentation and loss of self-worth. Nurses and other health-care professionals need to be aware of their patients' changing feelings with regard to body image and sexuality during a life-threatening and life-changing illness such as cancer.

References

Brennan J (2004) Cancer in Context: A practical guide to supportive care. Oxford: Oxford University Press.

Corner J, Bailey C (eds) (2001) Cancer Nursing Care in Context. Oxford: Blackwell.

Mick J, Hughes M, Cohen MZ (2004) Using the BETTER model to assess sexuality. Clin J Oncol Nurs 8(1): 84–6.

Nevidjon BM, Sowers KW (eds) (2000) A Nurse's Guide to Cancer Care. Philadelphia, PA: Lippincott.

Price B (1990) Body Image: Nursing concepts and care. London: Prentice Hall.

Quinn B (2003) Sexual health in cancer care. Nurs Times 99(4): 32–4.
Shell JA (1995) Do you like the things that life is showing you? The sensitive self-image of the person with cancer. Oncol Nurs Forum 22: 907–11.
Van Der Riet P (1998) The sexual embodiment of the cancer patient. Nurs Inquiry 5: 248–57.

Chapter 12

Legal and ethical issues

The focus of this chapter is exploration of the legal and ethical issues that may confront those caring for individuals with cancer. The chapter is not exhaustive; it discusses the issues of informed consent, confidentiality and truth telling, and advance statements (living wills). The more interested reader is directed to the many texts on ethics and legal issues for more in-depth information.

Informed consent

Consent derives from the Latin word *consentire*, which means to think or feel together (Faulder 1985), and the word informed means that information has been given. The giving of information does not, however, mean than the recipient necessarily understands this knowledge.

In the UK, nurses have a responsibility to ensure that patients in their care are given information about their condition and understand the risks and implications of any interventions required. The Nursing and Midwifery Council's *Code of Professional Conduct* (NMC 2002) states that clients have a right to receive information about their condition. *The Patient's Charter* (Department of Health or DoH 1991) also gave patients rights by stating that they should be given a clear explanation of any treatment proposed, including any risks and any alternatives.

The nurse must also respect the wishes of those who refuse or are unable to receive information about their condition. They have a responsibility to gain the consent of their patients before they carry out any procedure or intervention (NMC 2002). Individuals can exercise their autonomous right to make decisions about their care only if they have information about the choices available and the potential consequences of each action hence the term 'informed consent'. Nurses need to respect a patient's autonomy, even if this could result in harm, unless a court order rules to the contrary. According to Lavery (2003), in practice this does not always happen and consent in many cases is simply assumed. Faulder (1985) argues that most people, including doctors and patients, do not have a clear idea what informed consent is despite its importance. For consent to be given voluntarily it should be given freely and in the absence of distress (Cable 2003)

A brief history of informed consent

Informed consent has been a requirement in medical practice for more than two centuries (Aveyard 2002) and, in 1914, Judge Cardoza made the following statement after giving judgement in a case:

> Every human being of adult years and sound mind has a right to determine what shall be done with his own body and a surgeon who performs an operation without his patient's consent commits an assault, for which he is liable for damages.
>
> Gorovitz (In Aveyard 2002, p. 243)

The NMC's (2002) guidance for the nurse says that the every patient or client is legally competent unless otherwise assessed by a suitably qualified practitioner. The British Medical Association (BMA 1993) states that there are few conditions that necessarily prevent patients from giving informed consent. In the past there has been a belief that certain categories of patients, such as those with severe learning disabilities, are unable to give informed consent; however, Cable (2003) argues that it is the responsibility of the nurse to provide the time, information and support to enable the individual to make decisions. Only in extreme circumstances, where life is threatened, may the nurse act without consent (NMC 2002). Aveyard (2002) states that a response to the human experimentation that took place during World War II was that a set of principles relating to informed consent and clinical research was developed and the Nuremberg Code 1947 (1949) devised.

Properly informed?

To be properly informed, patients or research participants have a right to know exactly to what it is they are giving consent. Having this information should enable them to make a decision about a proposed intervention.

If the patient agrees to be part of a clinical trial the rules for information giving are more stringent. The Declaration of Helsinki (1975) details the ethical requirements for medical research and defines the parameters within which researchers may operate. In brief the declaration demands that practitioners ensure (Cable 2003):

- concern that the interest of the individual prevails over the interests of society or science
- that the individual is fully informed and aware that he or she can withdraw from the study at any time
- where there is any dependent relationship between practitioner and patients, that consent should be obtained by another practitioner who is not engaged in the research.

Is it ever possible for a patient to be fully informed?

The amount of information to be provided depends on the treatment or procedure. Usher and Arthur (1998) suggest that information and explanations on the following should be included in the information giving: the proposed treatment or procedure, which should be discussed together with possible risks and side effects, expected benefits, possible alternatives and the right to withdraw consent at any time. The consequences of no treatment should also be explained. The amount of information that a patient wishes to receive will vary. The Department of Health (2001) states that we should assume that the patient wishes to be well informed.

Nurse's role

The health-care services are increasingly subject to litigation and so it is essential that the principles of informed consent are understood by health-care workers. Patients and research participants should be fully informed about interventions and the information should be given in such a way as to facilitate understanding and decision-making. Nurses should be aware of the legal and professional requirements within which they work and remember that consent is required for all aspects of care, however minor. Failure to do this could mean that they face legal or disciplinary action.

Confidentiality

As discussed previously it is generally accepted that a person has a right to control access to his or her body. It is also accepted that he or she also has a right to control access to information about him- or herself. Patients grant access to their bodies and personal information about themselves on the understanding that access and information will be used for their benefit (Randall and Downie 1996). If patients feel that their confidentiality will be broken they may be unwilling to divulge important information that could harm their care (Gelling 1999). Rules about confidentiality have been present in medical ethics from the time of Hippocrates and are well established in the codes of practice of health professionals.

The NMC's *Code of Professional Conduct* (2002) states that information about patients and clients should be treated as confidential and used only for the purposes for which it was given. Patients and clients should understand that some information should be made available to other members of the team involved in the delivery of care. This information should be given to staff on a 'need to know' basis and is morally justifiable (Randall and Downie 1996). In the field of cancer care practitioners may work with trainees. Patients should be asked whether they consent to the trainee having access to confidential information and their wishes should be respected. Many patients seem to agree with the sharing of many aspects of information with their own close relatives and spouses. According to Randall and Downie (1996), however, it is not safe to assume that the patient agrees. Sometimes relatives are told a diagnosis before a competent patient is informed and in these cases a serious breach of confidentiality has occurred. Although they argue that many patients do not resent this because they wish their relatives to be told, the professional carers are not morally entitled to disclose this information to the relatives without the patient's permission. The duty of confidentiality is not dependent on patient autonomy and the duty applies in the non-autonomous patient. Confidentiality also applies to the deceased.

The duty of confidentiality is not absolute and in certain exceptional circumstances breaches of confidentiality are morally justifiable (Randall and Downie 1996). The NMC's *Code of Professional Conduct* (2002) states that disclosures where consent is either withheld or cannot be obtained is allowed only where they can be justified in the public interest either to protect an individual from harm or when required by law or order of a court.

Confidentiality and research

Upholding confidentiality in research is very important yet it is argued that, if disclosure of information from clinical records were not allowed, much research would not take place (McKane and Tolson 2000). As patients have the right to expect that their clinical records within the NHS are regarded as confidential, it seems obvious that they should be informed about where the information gained from research will be used

(DoH 1996). They should then be given the opportunity to opt out if they so wish (Pelham 1997). The Caldicott Committee Report (Caldicott 1997) urged that action be taken to increase awareness of the 1996 Department of Health guidance. Each health authority, NHS trust and primary care trust now has Caldicott guardians in place to protect the confidentiality of patient data (McKane and Tolson 2000).

Everything that health-care staff learn in the context of their professional relationship with patients should be regarded as confidential. The rules of confidentiality apply to non-autonomous and deceased patients as well as to autonomous patients. The information should be used only for the purpose for which it was given and not divulged to others without the patient's consent. In exceptional cases, where harm may be done to patients or others or when required by law or a court, information may be divulged where consent has not been given.

Truth telling

> No news is not good news it is an invitation to fear.
>
> Fletcher (1980, p. 994)

Health-care professionals often censor their information giving to patients in an attempt to protect them from potentially hurtful, sad or bad news (Fallowfield et al. 2002). Literature indicates that nurses have not come to terms with dealing with patients who have received bad news. Fallowfield et al. (2002) believe that this practice is present at all stages of cancer care. A common reason for not giving the news is that most patients do not wish to hear the truth because they will lose hope, become depressed and not enjoy their remaining time. In fact the opposite is true; in western Europe and North America the highest numbers of cases of depression are found in those not told the truth of their condition (Hall et al. 1996). There is also significant evidence from other parts of the world to suggest that many patients do not want cancer information disclosure and the usual practice is for doctors to disclose such information to the patient's family (Uchitomi and Yamawaki 1997). Often carers tell the family before the patients presumably because they find it easier to tell them. Some carers say that they want to talk to relatives first to ascertain the patient's best interests. Randall and Downie (1996) say that this is not a good-enough justification for telling the relatives first and, in the case of competent patients, the wishes of the relatives are not morally relevant. It is commonly thought that what people do not know does not harm them;

however, protecting patients from situations usually causes them more difficulties and a conspiracy of silence can lead to more fear, anxiety and confusion. Denying patients information takes away the opportunities to adapt and set achievable goals.

Doctors worldwide seriously underestimate the information needs of their patients (Fielding and Hung 1996); a recent study showed that most patients with cancer in the UK wanted all possible information, be it good or bad (Jenkins et al. 2001). Randall and Downie (1996) say that patients should be told as much of the truth as they want to know. There is very little available evidence that those with terminal illness who have not been told the truth of their situation die happy. Keeping the truth from a patient is difficult and others in the know will find it hard not to give out non-verbal clues about what is happening. Giving patients honest information will allow them to plan, put their affairs in order and say their goodbyes.

There is overwhelming evidence that imparting information related to the diagnosis of cancer is extremely stressful for both patients (Costello 1995, Morton 1996) and health-care professionals (Fallowfield 1993, Rosser 1994). The psychological and physical well-being of the patient can be affected and the health-care professional can be left feeling stressed and guilty. Staff and patients should therefore be supported through the event (Deeny and McGuigan 1999).

Research and truth telling

The research principle of veracity highlights the obligation of the researcher to tell the truth about the research study (Garity 1995). Telling the truth may deter potential participants from entering the study, yet it should still be told (Parahoo 1997). If researchers are not truthful or open they could withhold information about the study from the participant or raise false hope.

Advance statements (living wills)

Advance statements are living wills; they are an attempt to allow mentally competent adults to state, in advance, the kind of health care that they would authorize for themselves if at a future date they were unable to choose (Royal College of Nursing or RCN 1994). Individuals may discuss their preferences about being given a certain treatment. It can also include instructions for refusing treatment. This is often referred to as an advance directive. The sorts of treatments commonly listed in advance directives are artificial hydration and nutrition, mechanical ventilation and antibiotic therapy (Rashid 2000). Nurses are likely to be increasingly involved in discussing advance statements with patients who should be encouraged to review and update their advance statements from time to time because what might seem unacceptable in full health is sometimes actively requested in advanced disease (Gilbert 1996). Although the rights of patients are paramount, the patient does not have a right to refuse 'basic' care that health-care professionals always have a duty to provide. The BMA (1999) say that doctors should respect a patient's advance refusal of treatment made while mentally capable. The main concerns for nurses are: when to follow an advance statement, counselling patients before making an advance statement and the conscientious objection of colleagues (Rashid 2000).

Under new proposals published by the government in June 2003, people who fear that they will become mentally incapacitated would be able to appoint someone to ask doctors to stop life-sustaining treatment. The draft bill will make a type of 'living will' recognized in statute for the first time. Patients with debilitating diseases will be able to give 'lasting powers of attorney' to a family member or friend. The draft mental incapacity bill will affect the 2 million adults in the UK who are at some point unable to make decisions for themselves as a result of disability or mental illness. If the agreement is drawn up specifically to say so, consent can be refused for the doctors to give artificial nutrition. The Mental Capacity Bill was due to be discussed in Parliament in the summer of 2004. On 18 June 2004 the *Daily Mail* (see www.dailymail.co.uk/pages) stated that ministers were publishing the Mental Capacity Bill, which appeared in draft form last year.

Conclusion

This chapter has endeavoured to look briefly at some of the key ethical and legal issues that health-care professionals may face when caring for those with a life-threatening illness.

The study of ethics is not easy and professionals may face ethical issues on a daily basis. Ethics is central to all that we do. Although some might believe that it is only the major issues such as withdrawal of life-sustaining treatment and euthanasia that present ethical dilemmas, as discussed in this chapter the issues of confidentiality, information giving and consent, which may present themselves on a more frequent basis, also require attention. The legal position on issues such as advanced directives is changing and the reader is advised to consult the press for up-to-date information on the Mental Capacity Bill as it makes its way through parliament.

References

Aveyard H (2002) The requirement for informed consent prior to nursing care procedures. J Adv Nurs 39: 201–8.

BMA (1993) Medical Ethics Today: Its practice and philosophy. London: BMJ Publishing Group.

BMA (1999) Withholding and Withdrawing Life: Prolonging medical treatment: Guidance for decision making. London: BMJ Books.

Cable C (2003) Informed consent. Nurs Stand 18(12): 47–53.

Caldicott F (1997) Report of the Review of Patient Identifiable Information. London: DoH.

Costello J (1995) Helping relatives cope with the grieving process. Prof Nurse 11(2): 89–92.

Deeny K, McGuigan M (1999) The value of the nurse-patient relationship in the care of cancer patients. Nurs Stand 13(33): 45–7.

Department of Health (1991) The Patient's Charter. London: HMSO.

Department of Health (1996) Guidance on the Protection and Use of Patient's Information. London: HMSO.

Department of Health (2001) Good Practice in Consent Implementation Guide: www.doh.gov.uk/consent/implementationguide.pdf.

Fallowfield L (1993) Giving sad and bad news. Lancet 341: 476–8.

Fallowfield LJ, Jenkins VA, Beveridge HA (2002) Truth may hurt but deceit hurts more: communication in palliative care. Palliative Med 16: 297–303.

Faulder C (1985) Whose Body Is It? The troubling issue of informed consent. London: Virago.

Fielding RG, Hung J (1996) Preferences for information and involvement in decisions during cancer care among a Hong Kong Chinese population. Psycho-Oncology 5: 321–9.

Fletcher C (1980) Listening and talking to patients. BMJ 281: 994.

Garity J (1995) Ethics in research. In: Talbot LA (ed.), Principles and Practice of Nursing Research. St Louis, MO: Mosby.

Gelling L (1999) Ethical principles in health care research. Nurs Stand 13(36): 39–42.

Gilbert J (1996) The benefits and problems of living wills. Progr Palliative Care 4(1): 4–6.

Gorovitz S (ed) (1983) Moral Problems in Medicine, 2nd edn. Englewood Cliffs, NJ: Prentice Hall.

Hall A, Fallowfield LJ, A'Hern RP (1996) When breast cancer recurs: a 3 year prospective study of psychological morbidity. Breast J 2: 197–203.

Jenkins V, Fallowfield L, Saul J (2001) Information needs of patients with cancer: results from a large study in UK cancer centres. Br J Cancer 84: 48–51.

Lavery I (2003) Peripheral intravenous cannulation and patient consent. Nurs Stand 26(17): 10–42.

McKane M, Tolson D (2000) Research, ethics and the data protection legislation. Nurs Stand 14(20): 36–41.

Morton R (1996) Breaking bad news to patients with cancer. Cancer Nurs 11: 669–71.

Nuremberg Code 1947 (1949) Trials of War Criminals before the Nuremberg Military Tribunals under Control Council Law, vol. 10(2). Washington DC: US Government Printing Office, pp. 182–2.

Nursing and Midwifery Council (2002) Code of Professional Conduct. London: NMC.

Parahoo K (1997) Nursing Research: Principles, processes and issues. London: Macmillan

Pelham J (1997) Confidentiality, Implied Consent and Common Law. Edinburgh: Protec.

Randall F, Downie RS (1996) Palliative Care Ethics: A good companion. Oxford: Oxford University Press.

Rashid C (2000) Philosophical implications of the use of advance statements (living wills). Nurs Stand 14(25): 37–40.
Rosser MC (1994) The problems of denial. J Cancer Care 3(1): 12–17.
Royal College of Nursing (1994) Living Wills: Guidance for nurses. London: RCN.
Uchitomi Y, Yamawaki S (1997) Truth-telling practice in cancer care in Japan. In: Surobone A, Zwitter M (eds), Communication with the Cancer Patient. New York: New York Academy of Sciences, p. 809.
Usher K, Arthur D (1998) Process consent: a model for enhancing informed consent in mental health nursing. J Adv Nurs 27: 692–7.

Chapter 13

Surviving cancer

Living with cancer

Improved health promotion and treatments for cancer have contributed to earlier detection and increased chances of survival. Some long-term cancer survivors have a normal life expectancy and others, although not cured, live for a long time with cancer. For some cancers, the treatments needed to control the disease are intensive; for others a 'wait and see' policy can intensify the psychological trauma of living with a life-threatening illness. Survival of cancer should be accompanied by an acceptable quality of life for the individual. The trauma of a life-threatening illness and the almost unrecognizable life change are exasperated by our incapacity as a society to address, accept and communicate openly about the fear of our own mortality, which underlies cancer (Petrone 1999).

Problems commonly identified as long-term effects of cancer treatment include:

- fear of death
- fear of recurrence
- a preoccupation with health
- physical problems including fatigue, pain and long-term side effects of treatments
- psychological problems including anxiety and depression
- relationship difficulties.

Rehabilitation in cancer care involves adapting to changing circumstances over time and includes four aims:

1. Prevention: involves care aimed at preventing potential long-term problems, e.g. body image problems after mastectomy for breast cancer.
2. Restoration: returning the patient to a pre-cancer level of function. This might be physically possible but the patient may have psychological difficulties in returning.
3. Support: involves helping patients to adapt to long-term symptoms.
4. Palliation: this involves reducing the side effects of the disease process and treatment, and offering comfort and emotional support.

Several factors will influence individual coping styles, including:

- The nature of the cancer: type, site, extent
- Individual characteristics: age, gender, education, culture, religion, health beliefs
- Family characteristics: roles, responsibilities, communication, relationships, culture and values
- Support network characteristics: availability, flexibility, culture.

The role of the multidisciplinary team is key to supporting patients living with cancer, working together with the patient and the family to promote optimal quality of life – a quality of life that at times measures the difference between the hopes and expectations of an individual and that individual's experiences.

Hope

Many people react to a cancer diagnosis by preparing for death and, no matter what the prognosis, cancer forces people to examine the possibility that they may not live as long as they had thought (Brennan 2004). Suddenly hopes and dreams for the future are threatened, long-standing life goals become clear and at the same time their attainment may seem unlikely and even unrealistic.

Having things to look forward to and goals to achieve is what motivates and structures our lives; the threat of cancer leads people to re-evaluate life's hopes and dreams. Everyone needs a sense of hope and having hope involves more than just the wish to be cured. Having goals and plans, even if they are treatment related or even if they are made on a daily basis, are vital to people's sense of hope and meaning (Brennan 2004). The health-care professional who works with the patient and offers hope also enriches the life of the patient living with cancer.

Spirituality

Holistic care is based on the physical, psychosocial and spiritual needs of the individual. The multidisciplinary team works hard to meet the biopsychosocial needs of the patient, but often spiritual care is ignored, resulting in a failure to meet the spiritual pain, conflict and needs of the patient.

Patients with cancer experience loss, pain, fear, despair and often quote 'a search for meaning' or purpose for their life. Spirituality and a search for meaning are diverse concepts and encompass an individual's beliefs and values. Spiritual care can impact on the ability of patients to cope with a diagnosis of cancer, as well as subsequent treatments, providing a sense of purpose and meaning to life as well as preparation for death.

Nursing interventions that 'enspirit' people affected by cancer include:

- giving encouragement
- being quietly and professionally confident
- demonstrating genuine respect for the patient
- remembering the special characteristics of the patient in order to offer individualized care
- trusting the wisdom of struggling, standing by through the experience and protecting personal space and privacy
- being honest and open
- encouraging patients to talk about how they feel.

For some patients, confrontation with death results in a clarification of their understanding of human existence (Kinghorn and Gamlin 2001):

> If there is any place that needs any spirituality, it's here. If there's a place that needs God's kindness, it's here. . . . Because you're at your end. Some of them are going to die. Some of them are not going to die, but still, in this time of life, you need someone to be able to be kind and show God's love. Because otherwise it would be hell. . . . I couldn't stand to be here that many days without some kindness.
>
> Taylor (2003, p. 590)

Communication

Nurses are in the privileged position of being able to listen to patients talking about their hopes and fears related to their illness. The nurse's experience, knowledge and skills can enable patients and families to explore their feelings and adjust in some way to the situation; this may include discussing the situation openly or by using strategies such as humour or even avoidance in order for the individual to cope (Dean 2002).

It should be remembered that 'social talk' is also necessary; chatting and joking in a way that people take for granted may help to foster the hope that the illness has not taken over the patient's life entirely (Dean 2002, Wilkinson et al. 2002). Research evidence supporting *The NHS Cancer Plan* (DoH 2000) highlighted communication skills and the willingness to listen and explain as essential attributes of the health-care professional working in cancer care, along with sensitivity, approachability, respect and honesty, according to a national patient survey. Some patients went on to say that they received excellent care, with sensitive and thoughtful communication, clear information about their disease and its treatment, and good support when needed (DoH 2000). Other patients reported being given bad news in a deeply insensitive way, being left in the dark about their condition and being badly informed about their treatment and care. Complaints by patients focus not on a lack of competence but more often on the perceived failure of communication and an inability to convey a sense of care adequately (Wilkinson et al. 2002). According to Petrone (1999, p. 5):

> As a community we fail to realise that one lives through illness . . . as an individual the feelings that manifest in us are in fact because we are alive. The feelings of fear, pain, disbelief and anger only give more importance to the feelings of love, happiness and the value of life. . . . Who does not find it difficult to talk to someone who might be dying? The person assumes an aura of fragility that cannot afford a mistake. We are all human, we all make mistakes, how else do we learn and go forward?

Palliative care

> Sometimes the possibility of dying, gives permission for a way of living not previously allowed.
>
> Petrone (1999, p. 5)

Over 230 000 people in England and Wales will develop cancer each year, and cancer accounts for a quarter of all deaths. The diagnosis of cancer and its subsequent treatment can have a devastating impact not only on the individual's quality of life but also on the lives of their families and carers. Patients will face having to undergo unpleasant treatment options and they and their families and carers will need access to support from the time that the cancer is first suspected, through all stages of treatment to recovery, or in some cases to death and bereavement (National Institute for Clinical Excellence or NICE 2004).

Research has consistently shown that, in addition to receiving the best possible treatment, patients want and expect to be treated as individuals with dignity and with respect for their culture, lifestyles and beliefs. They want to have their voice heard and be able to exercise real choice about treatments and services. Patients want to receive detailed high-quality information about their condition and possible treatment and to be aware of the options available to them within the NHS, and the voluntary and independent sectors, including access to self-help groups and complementary therapy services (Cancerlink 2000).

Definition of palliative care

Palliative care is:

> The active holistic care of patient with advanced progressive illness. Management of pain and other symptoms and provision of psychological, social and spiritual support is paramount. The goal of palliative care is achievement of the best quality of life for patients and their families. Many aspects of palliative care are also applicable earlier in the course of the illness in conjunction with other treatments.
>
> World Health Organization (WHO 2002)

Palliative care principles

Palliative care is based on a number of principles and has a number of aims:

- To provide relief from pain and other distressing symptoms.
- To integrate the psychological and spiritual aspects of patient care.
- To offer a support system to help patients to live as actively as possible until death and to help the family to cope during the patient's illness and in their own bereavement.
- To be applied early in the course of illness in conjunction with other therapies intended to prolong life (National Council for Hospice and Specialist Palliative Care Services or NCHSPCS 2002, WHO 2002).

Palliative care is recognized in *The NHS Cancer Plan* (DoH 2000) as having a crucial role in the care received by patients and carers throughout the course of their disease. It states that too many patients still experience distressing symptoms, poor nursing care, poor psychological and social support, and inadequate communication from health-care professionals during the final stages of an illness, and it calls for the care of dying patients to improve to the level of the best (DoH 2000).

Palliative care can be provided by those who care for patients on a day-to-day basis; until recently it was categorized as the palliative care approach and has now been redefined as general palliative care (NCHSPCS 2002). Specialist palliative care is delivered by those who specialize in palliative care, e.g. consultants in palliative medicine and clinical nurse specialists (NCHSPCS 2002). The document *Palliative Care in the Hospital*

Setting (NCHSPCS 1996) recommended that the palliative care approach should be an integral part of all clinical practice and should be available to all patients with life-threatening illness. Much of the professional support given to patients with advanced cancer is given by professionals who are not specialists and may have received little training in this area. The NICE (2004) recommends that medical and nursing services are available for patients with advanced cancer on a 24-hour, 7-days-a-week basis, and specialist advice should be available at all times. Staff should receive training and ensure that they have the knowledge and skills needed for their role.

Supportive care

The NICE (2004), in a recent publication, discusses the importance of supportive care, stating that although it is not a distinct speciality it is the responsibility of all health-care and social care professionals. It involves open and sensitive communication. Supportive care begins when the patient is first seen. The NCHSPCS (2002, p. 3) says that supportive care:

> . . . helps the patient and their family cope with cancer and its treatment from pre-diagnosis through diagnosis and treatment, to cure, continuing illness or death and into bereavement. It helps the patient maximise the benefits of treatment and to live as well as possible with the effects of the disease. It is given equal priority alongside diagnosis and treatment.

Although the palliative care and supportive care definitions are very similar it is useful to have supportive care defined in order that patients and families can have an idea of the type of care and support that they can expect.

There is both a growing interest and need to expand the provision of palliative care to those with diseases other than cancer. In doing so the potential to relieve suffering is increased.

Conclusion

Supportive care for those people living with cancer whether after curative treatment, during active treatment or in the terminal stages of disease should be addressed by all members of the multidisciplinary team. It is important that the cancer patient has goals and plans; these might be short or long term or even on a daily basis; they might be treatment related or even psychosocial or emotional (Brennan 2004). The physical, psychosocial and spiritual needs of the patient should be embraced by health-care professionals working in partnership with the patient and his or her family (NICE 2004).

For those patients where treatment is no longer available and no cure possible, and where health-care professionals understand the meaning of the illness for the patient and that patient's life, there is a sense of healing – in the sense that by understanding the meaning of the illness the patient can overcome the sense of alienation, loss of self-understanding and loss of social integration that can accompany illness. For the health-care professional who is involved in the support of the patient with cancer, involvement and caring can lead to loss and pain; however, it can also make joy and fulfilment possible (Benner and Wrubel 1989).

References

Benner P, Wrubel J (1989) The Primacy of Caring: Stress and coping in health and illness. Los Angeles, CA: Addison-Wesley.

Brennan J (2004) Cancer in Context: A practical guide to supportive care. Oxford: Oxford University Press.

Cancerlink (2000) Cancer Supportive Care Services Strategy: Users' priorities and perspectives. London: Cancerlink.

Dean A (2002) Talking to dying patients of their hopes and needs. Nurs Times 98(3): 34–5.

Department of Health (2000) The NHS Cancer Plan: A plan for investment, a plan for reform. London: HMSO.

Kinghorn S, Gamlin R (2001) Palliative Nursing: Bringing comfort and hope. Oxford: Baillière Tindall.

National Council for Hospice and Specialist Palliative Care Services (1996) Palliative Care in the Hospital Setting. Occasional Paper no. 10. London: NCHSPCS.

National Council for Hospice and Specialist Palliative Care Services (2002) Definitions of Supportive and Palliative Care. Briefing Paper no. 11. London: NCHSPCS.

National Institute for Clinical Excellence (2004) Guidance on Cancer Services. Improving supportive and palliative care for adults with cancer. The Manual. London: NICE.

Petrone M (1999) Touching the Rainbow: Pictures and words by people affected by cancer. East Sussex: Brighton and Hove Health Promotion Department.

Taylor EJ (2003) Nurses caring for the spirit: patients with cancer and family caregiver expectations. Oncol Nurs Forum 30: 585–90.

Wilkinson SM, Gambles M, Roberts A (2002) The essence of cancer care: the impact of training on nurse's ability to communicate effectively. J Adv Nurs 40: 731–8.

World Health Organisation (2002) National Cancer Control Programmes: Policies and guidelines. Geneva: WHO.

Index